# DR SEBI BIBLE
# 14 IN 1

THE ULTIMATE GUIDE TO DETOX AND CLEANSE YOUR BODY NATURALLY
WHILE BOOSTING YOUR IMMUNE SYSTEM. LIVE A DISEASE-FREE LIFE
WITH DR. SEBI'S APPROVED ALKALINE REMEDIES & METHODS

JUDITH CARLSON

# TABLE OF CONTENTS

# DR. SEBI DIET

## ABOUT DR. SEBI

The man behind the Dr. Sebi Diet is Alfredo Bowman. He is a Honduran self-proclaimed herbalist and healer who uses food to improve health. Although he is already deceased, he has many followers in the 21st century. He has claimed to cure many diseases using herbs and a strict vegan diet because of his holistic approach. He has set up a treatment center in his home country before moving to New York City, where he has continued his practice and extended his clienteles from Michael Jackson, John Travolta, Eddie Murphy, and Steven Sea gal, to name a few.

Although he calls himself Dr. Sebi, he does not hold any medical nor Ph.D. degree. Moreover, the diet has claimed to cure different conditions such as sickle-cell anemia, lupus, leukemia, and HIV-AIDS. That led to a lot of issues, particularly that he was practicing medicine without a license. While he was charged for practicing without a license, he was acquitted in the early 1990s due to a lack of evidence. However, he was instructed to stop making claims that his diet can treat HIV-AIDS. While controversies surround his name, there are so many benefits of his alkaline vegan diet that it is still popular even to this date.

Dr. Sebi believed that acidity and mucus could cause different types of diseases. For instance, the build-up of mucus in the lungs can lead to pneumonia. He noted that eating certain food types and avoiding others like the plague can help detoxify the body. It can also bring the body to an alkaline state that can reduce the risk of developing many diseases. By turning the blood alkaline, the cells can be rejuvenated and can easily eliminate toxins out. Moreover, he argues that diseases cannot exist in an environment that is alkaline.

This particular diet relies on eating a list of approved foods and certain types of supplements. For the body to heal itself, Dr. Sebi noted that this diet should be followed consistently for the rest of your life.

Here is a compiled list of what differentiates the Dr. Sebi Diet from a plant-based diet:

- No processed foods: Tofu, veggie burgers, textured vegetable protein, canned fruits, canned vegetables, oil, soy sauce, and other condiments are considered processed. The Dr. Sebi Diet encourages dieters to consume unadulterated food. Some plant-based diets still allow processed foods as long as they are made from plant-based ingredients.
- No wheat products allowed: Under this diet regimen, you are not allowed to consume wheat and wheat products such as bread, biscuits, and others as they are not naturally growing grains. Naturally growing grains include amaranth seeds, wild rice, and triticale, to name a few.
- The need to adhere to the food list: In general, plant-based diets are not so restrictive when it comes to the food that dieters can eat (unless you are specifically following a strict plant-based

regimen such as the plant-based keto diet). However, the Dr. Sebi Diet requires dieters only to eat foods listed in the nutritional guide.

- Drink one (1) gallon of water daily: Water is the most hydrating liquid on the planet. The Dr. Sebi Diet requires dieters to consume 1 gallon of water daily or more. Moreover, tea and coffee should be avoided as these drinks are highly acidic.
- Taking in Dr. Sebei's supplements: If you are taking any medications for a particular health condition, this particular diet regimen will require you to consume proprietary supplements an hour before taking your medication.

## Dr. Sebi Teaching and Methods

Dr. Sebi classified food into six categories:

1. Drugs
2. Genetically modified foods
3. Hybrid foods
4. Dead foods
5. Living foods
6. Raw foods

He concluded that the first four categories of food in this list are no go area as they cause more body damage than good. These foods can cause a build-up of acids and mucus in the body. However, the last two categories of foods are the best types of food he classified as healthy because the nutritional contents in them are not lost in any way. For instance, foods that are thoroughly cooked, hybridized, and modified have lost the required amount of nutrients present in them. Hence, instead of providing benefits for the body, the reverse is the case. However, raw foods, especially vegetables, fruits, and herbs, are excellent for building good health.

Dr. Sebi's diet is a plant-based and electric diet based on the 'African bio-mineral' that helps dieters fight diseases. The diet also serves to prevent various diseases (prophylaxis) and boost the immune system. When the body is immuno-compromised, it is said to accommodate any infection that sneaks in.

Dr. Sebi's diet is also beneficial for people who cherish to live a healthy life by remaining clean and lean. His diet was not created from heaven; they are common foods we ignore because of the love of modified, processed, refined, and hybridized foods.

Dr. Sebi's diet contains vegetables, fruits, grains, nuts, herbal teas, plant-based sweeteners, and seeds. Those who cherish animal products will not benefit from this diet as it does not encourage foods made from animals.

According to Dr. Sebi, all infections grow well in the environment that makes them comfortable such as acidic, mucus overload, and toxic environs.

When the body is in a limy condition, infections will find it so difficult to thrive, and when it is in an acidic state, the reverse is the case. Hence, the acidic component in the body helps diseases to multiply and thrive.

Likewise, he also declared that the build-up of excess mucus in the body increases the susceptibility of having an infection as the mucus block up the blood vessel and easily hinders blood flow.

He stated that the excess mucus must be removed for you to enjoy your health. When the mucus is removed either by detoxification or cleansing, the diseases are automatically removed.

The healing of many sufferers who suffer from hair loss and many other prevalent diseases didn't occur because of the medications they took but because of the self-healing that took place in the body due to Dr. Sebi's alkaline diet.

This diet is rich in fibers, especially from whole grains and vegetables. Fibers are beneficial in that they help deal with constipation and ease bowel movements.

Limiting ultra-processed foods improves the quality of the diet in the overall scheme of things.

## COLLATERAL EFFECTS OF WESTERN MODERN MEDICINE IN CHRONIC DISEASES

The source of most major chronic diseases lies in the Western tradition of modern medicine and diet. Some of the oldest, such as heart disease, cancer, diabetes, and autoimmune disease are all very old diseases that have been around for hundreds to thousands of years before the advent of these practices. The main difference between now and then is due to collaterals from each individual being different based on a variety of socioeconomic factors. For example: Men typically have more thrombosis (blood clots) as compared to women since men are not significantly protected by estrogen during pregnancy giving them a higher risk factor for blood clots. Also, men have a greater risk of heart disease since they tend to have more risk factors for heart disease as compared to women. Today we are mainly responsible for consuming a diet that is lacking in essential vitamins, minerals and fats. This has led to a deficiency of essential nutrients causing the Western world public to suffer from the ill effects of modern medicine.

Using the vegetable oil based rather than animal fat based diet common during this time period; food has been processed and stored which has made it lose much of its nutritional value which is once again due to overpopulation due in part by excess livestock production. The soils in most developed countries are depleted because they are used as feed crops and not being replenished with additional nutrients. We live in a society where we are overfed and undernourished. There is an oversupply of food and a large deficiency in nutrients. This is the reason why we require vitamin and mineral supplements to correct a deficiency in our diet. The result has been an increase in chronic diseases that has led to a compromised immune system which uses up much of our body's resources to protect itself against such chronic diseases. We are living in an environment that is similar to conditions found during the bubonic plague with its high risk factors for developing major diseases, like cancer, coronary artery disease and heart attacks.

## HOW TO DETOX YOUR BODY

You look great, but you still feel awful, sluggish, and foggy. It's time to detox!

You may be wondering how to detox or what the benefits of detoxing are. Detoxing is a natural process your body does to clean out any potentially toxic substances that could inhibit your organs from performing correctly.

Detoxifying can include removing unwanted chemicals, candida, surface metals accumulated from eating acidic foods that keep the body in an inflammatory state, and other forms of waste, including fecal matter stored in the colon.

Detoxification is how cells can get rid of waste materials that may have built up in their system. We were told that you needed to consume more acidic foods to detoxify for years, but this is not true!

The human body is a complicated system, and it's difficult to imagine how any single food can be excellent or horrible for it. But that doesn't mean that some foods don't have more of an advantage than others.

Some people, however, think that returning the ph level in the body back to natural alkaline levels will help decrease inflammation. And while this does seem like something worth investigating because of all the benefits alkaline foods offer, like helping your digestion and providing powerful antioxidants for your immune system, there is no research backing up any specific diet as a "detox food."

The alkaline diet is the most popular detox diet. Alkaline foods are said to have a much more beneficial effect on the body than acidic foods. In many cases, a powerful alkaline diet will help improve various health conditions. If you think you might want to try an alkaline diet, we will give you the essential info about an alkaline diet and what food standards should be consumed.

This will show you how an alkaline diet and pH balance diet can help bring your body back into balance. You'll learn what foods are best for detoxing and how certain types of food can increase your energy levels as well as your physical health.

But why should I be detoxing, and how does it help me? After all, we are told that the body "cleans itself" naturally as our metabolism, water, and other fluids naturally flush toxins through our body.

The problem with this is that we have toxins in our bodies that are not being removed! Think about it. Have you ever had a drink and then felt like you were poisoned? This is the result of toxins in your system that are not being cleared. The toxins stay trapped inside your body, hurting you no matter how much water, exercise, or fruit you drink.

Are you dreaming about how great it will be to increase weight loss through detoxing? Well, first of all, we don't need to lose weight! Detoxing helps us get rid of waste and toxic materials.

It's essential to have a healthy lifestyle.

When you have an average pH level and a healthy diet, you feel good and look vibrant with shiny hair and glowing skin - not to mention all the energy you have!

When you adjust your pH to a healthier level, you experience a lasting quality of life. An alkaline diet can help repair areas in the body that have become damaged by oxidative stress or unhealthy nutrition. This is because body cells can repair themselves when the body is in balance and receive adequate nutrition. The main reason the alkaline diet is so effective is that it returns to your body's natural pH, somewhere around 7.35-7.45, which has been proven by science to be what your body can repair itself into naturally when there are no outside influences on its pH.

The pH diet: What you can eat

Before changing your diet, it is recommended that you check your pH balance with a saliva test kit or urinalysis - these can be purchased at any drugstore. When doing a saliva test, you need to have freshly drawn saliva because the saliva pH levels will change during the day and after eating. After you get a read on your pH, you can begin making changes.

The ideal food choices are those that are alkaline-forming. A food with a pH of 8 or higher is considered alkaline-forming, and those under pH 7 are acid-forming. You can eat plenty of fresh fruits and vegetables, whole grains, legumes, nuts, and seeds to your heart's content! However, meats are more challenging to digest, making them harder for the body to break down into smaller particles to be absorbed into the cells - the heart will cause a more acidic reaction in your body. Dairy products such as milk, cheese, and yogurt should also be avoided since they are considered acid-forming. However, yogurt is a better option than regular milk since it has probiotics that help restore your gut health.

The alkaline-forming foods include:

Vegetables: all leafy greens, like spinach and kale; broccoli; cauliflower; celery; cabbage; cucumber.

All leafy greens, like spinach and kale; broccoli; cauliflower; celery; cabbage; cucumber. Fruits: berries such as blueberries and blackberries are very alkaline-forming; peaches, mangos, apples, and pears are also excellent choices.

Berries such as blueberries and blackberries are very alkaline-forming; peaches, mangos, apples, and pears are also excellent choices. Grains: quinoa and amaranth are alkaline-forming grains that you can eat in moderation. Other grains, like wheat and corn, are acid-forming, so they should be eaten only in moderation or not at all.

Quinoa and amaranth are alkaline-forming grains that you can eat in moderation. Other grains, like wheat and corn, are acid-forming, so they should be eaten only in moderation or not at all. Legumes: all legumes, except for soybeans, are alkaline-forming.

All legumes, except for soybeans, are alkaline-forming. Nuts and seeds: almonds; peanuts; walnuts; sunflower seeds.

Almonds; peanuts; walnuts; sunflower seeds. Some examples include garlic, ginger root, cilantro, black pepper, and turmeric - which have anti-inflammatory effects on the body!

Herbs and spices contain a multitude of healing properties and are very alkaline-forming. Some examples include garlic, ginger root, cilantro, black pepper, and turmeric - which have anti-inflammatory effects on the body! Dairy products: milk, yogurt, and cheese should be avoided; instead, drink a glass of unsweetened almond milk to get the calcium you need.

Milk, yogurt, and cheese should be avoided; instead, drink a glass of unsweetened almond milk to get the calcium you need. Like any other non-vegetarian food, alcohol should be limited to no more than two drinks per day.

As with any other non-vegetarian food, alcohol should be limited to no more than two drinks per day. Sugary foods: anything that is high in sugar should be avoided. This includes all processed foods and overly sweetened fruit juices. Instead, focus on eating whole fruits and vegetables - these will help to alkalize your body, but they are also a great source of vitamins, minerals, and fiber, which helps keep insulin levels low, which helps with weight loss!

Alkaline-forming foods can balance the body's pH levels by alkalizing the body, while acid-forming foods will acidify it. The ideal pH ranges for adults are between 6 and 7; this is what you want to aim for! To check your pH levels or some other considerations when it comes to diet, visit www.natural-healthybodyguide.com.

Your body is comprised of numerous components, and all must work together for you to live healthily at an optimal level. The digestive system, nervous system, and endocrine system - along with the liver and gallbladder - all work together daily to create a healthy life every day.

As is the case with most things - if the system is not working correctly, it won't be too long before we begin to feel sick and start having health issues. As a result, we need to balance our body's internal pH regularly to remain efficient at all times. Once we begin to get out of balance, we need to know how to get back to the correct pH to feel better. This is why it is so important to get yourself into an alkaline state regularly - and this is something that can be done in the comfort of your own home or at home with the help of a professional.

Are you acidified? The balance between alkalinity and acidity needs to be maintained for optimum health, which begins by understanding its pH balance.

In addition to dieting for better food selection, a whole-body approach includes healthy habits such as meditation or yoga – or any other way of managing stress levels. It's also essential to maintain proper hydration levels. Water is the key to alkalinity, and drinking enough water allows the body to function at its best.

We lose a lot of our water every day through breathing, sweating, and elimination through urination. If you have inadequate hydration, this can lead to acidity – a type of derangement that is very common in America today! The pH scale uses 0 to 14 to measure the acidity or alkalinity of substances. Normal pH levels range from 1-6; anything below 7 (acidic) or above 7 (alkaline) is considered unhealthy. Sugar and carbohydrates are both very sour, so a diet rich in these types of foods can lead to acidity.

How to detox with alkaline foods and pH balanced diet.

You can address acidity anywhere in your body with many different techniques, but there are two that stand out: alkaline foods and pH balanced diet. Both have been used as a natural way of detoxing for centuries. The alkaline food technique is the best way to begin the process of rebalancing the body's pH balance since it includes plenty of alkaline vegetables and fruits grown at higher pH levels.

Alkaline foods are grown in greenhouses, which are kept at a higher pH level. They often include apple juice, molasses, and Rumney Creek Mangosteen juice. These fresh alkaline foods work best against acidity, especially if you're not eating enough protein. It's best to start with an organic diet that doesn't contain sugar and processed carbohydrates. Remember to drink two big glasses of pure water every day – one at mealtime and the other before bedtime for best results!

The Differences Between an Alkaline Diet and Ph Balanced Diet

One of the main differences between an alkaline diet and a pH-balanced diet is that the former focuses on a minimal number of foods, while the latter offers lots of fresh fruits and vegetables to eat. The alkaline diet (permaculture) emphasizes using natural cultivation methods such as permaculture, aquaculture, mushroom growing, etc. This integrates the practices of healthy food cultivation into a lifestyle that avoids toxins in food and water.

The pH-balanced diet has taken the best aspects of the alkaline diet and added more natural whole foods with higher pH levels (pH 11- 12). Foods that are alkaline range from whole grain cereals to dark chocolate and even fruits and vegetables. This is a beautiful way to detox since it allows the body to eliminate toxins through the kidneys and bowels, which cannot do so.

## DR. SEBI SUPERFOODS

The super-foods listed below may not be available everywhere or may not be available throughout the year, but there are so many of them that regardless of where you live, or which time of the year it is, you are bound to have access to at least some of them.

15 Dr. Sebi Approved foods that help fight Diabetes:

1. All Leafy greens listed in Dr. Sebi Nutritional Guide

These are kale, lettuce (except iceberg), wild arugula, onions, etc. Leafy veggies are some of the most natural electric foods because they are loaded with minerals (Calcium, Iron, magnesium and potassium) and vitamins (C, K, E, and B vitamins).

2. Cherry or Plum Tomatoes

Tomatoes are a rich source of vitamins, particularly C, A, and K. What's more, a single tomato can provide about 40% of the daily recommended dose of vitamin C. It improves your vision, digestion, and skin. It's also rich in lycopene which helps reduce the risk of certain types of cancer, e.g. prostate, ovarian, lung, and stomach.

3. Avocado

This fruit is loaded with nutrients and can help improve many diabetes and pre-diabetes. Avocado is loaded with fiber which boosts friendly gut bacteria. Avocado is the food to eat if you undergo chemotherapy because it helps reduce side effects.

4. Olive oil

Cold-pressed olive oil is one of the best oils there is. It's rich in healthy fats that help reduce inflammation, contains a lot of antioxidants that protect you from diabetes, stroke and heart problems. It also has anti-cancer properties, relieves rheumatoid arthritis inflammation, and helps fight infections.

5. Berries

High in vitamins, minerals, and fiber, blueberries have the highest antioxidant level of all fruits. Regular consumption of these berries is one of the best protections against premature aging and cancer. Blueberries can prevent heart disease, improve cognitive performance, help with urinary tract infections, boost your eye health, and much more. Besides, by keeping your brain sharp, they indirectly protect you against Alzheimer's.

6. Key Lime

Lime is very rich in vitamin C and soluble fiber, a combination that helps protect you against diabetes and heart disease. It is also efficient protection against kidney stones, anemia, cancer, and various digestive problems.

7.  Apples

This popular fruit is so nutrient-dense, that eating them regularly lowers the risk of many diseases. Apples can stabilize blood glucose levels, reduce the risk of diabetes, maintain a healthy cholesterol level, and a healthy heart. Besides, an apple a day will improve your digestion, reduce the risk of certain types of cancer, diabetes, and stroke.

8.  Walnuts

Walnuts are super rich in omega-3s, and you should eat a dozen or so every day. If taken regularly, walnuts can easily reduce your cholesterol levels, improve insulin sensitivity, boost memory, and protect you against certain types of cancers.

## Foods you should never eat (and why)

Regardless of the diet you're on, there are usually foods you should eat more of, as well as those you should stay away from. Today, there are dozens of healthy, as well as fad diets, and they all have their "followers." However, there are some foods everyone should not only stay away from but avoid them like a plague. These foods are more than just unhealthy. Some of them contain so many artificial additives and synthetic chemicals, they are actually dangerous to eat.

Unfortunately, many of these foods are very popular and we eat them all the time. Some of them are even offered by health food shops. When you go through this list, you'll understand why the so-called diseases of civilization are becoming a serious threat to global health. Three things that most unhealthy foods have in common:

•  They are popular

Most of these foods are on our table every day. What's even worse, some of them are sold in health food shops as healthy alternatives to sugar, meat or dairy.

•  They are aggressively marketed

The meat and dairy industries have powerful lobbies that successfully manipulate people into buying foods they shouldn't. Aggressive marketing campaigns and misleading messages have resulted in consumers becoming unable to decide for themselves, but doing what they are told.

•  They are tasty, cheap, and convenient

What makes giving up these foods so difficult, is that most of them are very tasty (because they are full of flavor additives), cheap (because they are mass-produced from the cheapest ingredients), and convenient (many of them are pre-packed and ready to use, requiring minimum preparation time). The story of modern agriculture and the stressful sedentary lifestyle we now lead is a long and complicated one and is beyond the scope of this book. Suffice it to say that your diet should be much more than fuel that keeps you going.

A diet can be a source of healing or toxic foods. It can improve or destroy your health. It can boost your mood and performance or contribute to premature aging and chronic disease. So, whatever food you think is best for you, make sure it's free of the following foods:

1.  Canned foods

All canned foods contain Bisphenol A (BPA). This chemical is used in can lining and has been linked to infertility, obesity, cancer, and other conditions. Whenever possible, choose fresh or frozen foods instead of canned ones.

2.  Deep-fried foods

Deep-fried foods are usually very tasty which is why we love them. However, they are cooked in a lot of oil which makes them very fatty. Besides, what makes it even more unhealthy is that such oil is usually reused many times.

3.  Instant noodles

Instant noodles, just like all other instant foods, are full of preservatives, and color- and flavor additives. Besides, they contain a lot of calories and sodium. If you often eat instant noodles, you risk having a stroke, developing diabetes or succumbing to heart disease.

4.  Margarine

Margarine is based on trans fats. These clog arteries and restrict the flow of blood to the heart. When it first appeared on the market, we were told it was healthier than butter and would protect our hearts. Today, we know this is nonsense. Regular consumption of trans fats increases your risk of developing type 2 diabetes or heart disease.

5.  Soft drinks

Soft drinks contain a lot of sugar (about 40 grams per bottle) and if taken regularly will increase your blood sugar levels which can lead to many serious conditions, eg high blood pressure, diabetes, etc.

6.  Packaged Fruit juices

Many people start their day with a glass of orange juice. Well, they shouldn't. It takes four oranges to produce a single glass of juice. Although juice is a healthy beverage, unfortunately, all the fiber from the fruit has been discarded. Besides, fruit juice contains almost as much sugar as soft drinks. A better way to start a day would be to eat an orange, not drink a glass of orange juice. That way, you'll get all the vitamins, plus the fiber, and the amount of fructose your liver has to deal with would be minimal.

7.  Artificial sweeteners

Artificial sweeteners are found in many sugar-free products, et chewing gums, baked goods, jams, etc. They are also what sugar replacements are based on, e.g. xylitol, erythritol, isomalt, lactitol, maltitol, mannitol, sorbitol. Although these artificial sweeteners are marketed as natural, they are actually heavily processed and are often produced from GMO ingredients. Long-term use of artificial sweeteners can create an imbalance in your gut flora and contribute to the development of diabetes, gastrointestinal problems, weight gain, etc.

8.  Soy protein

Most of the soy produced in the US (as well as in some other countries) is genetically modified. The reason GM soy is now farmed is that it is resistant to glyphosate, a weedkiller commonly used in soy farming. A recent Norwegian study found that US-produced soy contains so much of this herbicide, it almost feels like you are eating weedkiller. Glyphosate is linked to many life-threatening conditions, including several types of lymphoma cancer. While fermented soy products, such as natto, tempeh, and miso soups are perfectly safe to use, you must stay away from edamame, soy milk, and soy protein.

9. Farmed salmon (Atlantic salmon)

Most people eat salmon because it's high in omega-3 fatty acids. However, farmed salmon available today have considerably lower levels of these healthy fats than the salmon we could buy only five years ago. The most likely reason for this is that salmon is now fed much less nutritious food. Besides, dioxin levels are ten times higher in farmed salmon than in wild salmon. This is bad news because this chemical is linked to cancer, organ damage, and immune system dysfunction.

On top of that, farmed salmon is regularly treated with banned pesticides. To make things even worse, it recently became legal to produce and sell genetically engineered salmon without having to label it as such.

10. Meat from large-scale farms

All animals raised this way are fed growth hormones, antibiotics, and food grown with chemical pesticides and fertilizers. A recent analysis of chicken meat and feathers discovered traces of banned antibiotics, allergy medications, painkillers, and even arsenic.

11. Microwave popcorn

The microwavable bags are lined with perfluorochemicals that make the bags resistant to heat. Unfortunately, these chemicals are linked to cancer. Besides, the fake butter flavoring that's often used in the production of popcorn is known to cause lung disease and inflammation in various organs.

12. Shrimp

Farmed shrimps contain a certain food additive that is used to improve the color of shrimp. This additive has estrogen-like effects that can affect the sperm count in men and increase the risk of breast cancer in women. Besides, ponds where shrimps are raised, are often treated with neurotoxic pesticides known to cause certain neurological problems, eg attention deficit symptoms, impaired memory, etc.

13. Table salt

Iodine is one of the most essential trace elements our body needs for proper functioning which is why we should use only iodized salt. Salt comes either from underground salt deposits or the sea. Although the natural salt is rich in minerals, by the time it is delivered to shops, it has been processed so much, that none of its original nutrients remain. Besides, salt rich in natural minerals is never white which is why it is bleached (to look clean). After bleaching, various anticaking agents are added to make it free-flowing. Excessive consumption of salt (including the mineral-rich healthy salt) increases the risk of high blood pressure, heart disease, stroke, kidney disease, etc.

14. Vegetable oils

Vegetable oils, e.g. canola, cottonseed, corn or soybean oil, are as bad as margarine. If you use a lot of oil or eat a lot of deep-fried foods, you will become more vulnerable to certain diseases, eg inflammation, atherosclerosis, certain types of cancer, diabetes, digestive disorders, heart disease, high cholesterol, liver problems, obesity, etc.

15. Fat-free and low-fat milk

When raw milk is pasteurized, it loses a lot of its nutrients. Long-life milk is particularly unhealthy because it first has to be dried at temperatures of about 1000 degrees Centigrade, after which water is added to it. Needless to say, no enzymes or any other nutrients can survive these high temperatures.

People usually choose low-fat or fat-free dairy products because they don't want to gain weight. However, what they don't realize is that when fat is removed, carbs or sugar are added. This is done so that milk would have flavor, otherwise, it would taste like water. So, fat-free and low-fat milk contains added sugar, which, if you drink a lot of milk, puts you at risk of developing diabetes or heart disease.

16. Coffee with added flavors

Black coffee has a number of health benefits and can even protect you from certain liver diseases. However, after sugar, whipped cream or powdered milk has been added to it, it becomes a very unhealthy beverage.

17. Seitan

We usually think of seitan as a healthy alternative to meat protein. However, it is simply wheat gluten. This means that even if you are not allergic to gluten but you often eat seitan, you may develop gluten intolerance symptoms. Besides, seitan contains a lot of sodium, over 500 milligrams per 100 grams.

It gets even more unhealthy if you add non-dairy liquid creamers based on corn syrup. Black coffee is the healthiest option because although these additives improve the taste of coffee, they also contribute to increased liver fat and some gastrointestinal problems.

18. Burnt food

Bunt foods should be avoided whenever possible. This is necessary partly because they are more difficult to digest, but especially because they produce cancer-causing chemicals. Burnt meat in particular is very unhealthy. Although many people find charred meat tastier than medium-to-rare, the risk of ingesting carcinogens is not worth the improved taste.

19. Diet soda

The main reason you should avoid diet soda is that it's full of artificial sweeteners. For a number of reasons, these are worse for your health than ordinary sugar. So, if you drink diet soda regularly, you are at a higher risk of developing both cancer and diabetes.

20. Processed meats

Many people can't imagine a sandwich without salami but cured meats are so full of saturated fat, sodium, and preservatives, that if you are into healthy eating, this is one of the first foods you should give up.

21. Canned green beans

For some reason, U.S.-grown canned green beans are some of the most toxic canned foods there are. This food is treated with some of the most dangerous pesticides and eating just one serving a day, puts you at risk of developing cancer and having other health problems. Besides, all cans are lined with materials that contain Bisphenol A. This is a synthetic estrogen that can create fertility problems for both men and women. Unless you can find fresh or frozen green beans, this is one of the foods you must avoid at all costs.

22. Non-organic strawberries

Some fruits and vegetables contain so many toxins from pesticides and fertilizers, that they are actually dangerous to eat. One of them is strawberries. Besides the pesticides, the soil on which non-organic strawberries are grown, is often treated with toxic gases. These were initially developed for chemical warfare, but are now used in agriculture. In other words, if you can't afford organic strawberries, stay away from them.

23. Energy drinks

The reason they are so addictive is that they taste so good. Which they do because they are full of sugar and flavor additives. Long-term use of energy drinks is linked to inflammatory processes, heart disease, and certain neurological problems.

The list of unhealthy foods is much longer but the bottom line is to try and stay away from all processed, instant or foods that don't even look like food. Whenever possible, stick to organically grown fruits and vegetables and grass-fed meat, dairy, and eggs.

24. Packaged foods

They are usually very tasty which is why we love them. However, they are cooked in a lot of oil which makes them very fatty. Besides, what makes it even more unhealthy is that such oil is usually reused many times.

## COMMON BUT DANGEROUS ILLNESSES YOU CAN TREAT WITH THIS DIET

Hypertension

High blood pressure and Hypertension is a long-term health problem in which blood pressure is gradually rising. It is a significant risk factor for strokes, heart disease, vision loss, and even dementia. To be healed, we must keep away from meat and alcohol, drink not too much tea, and eat fruits and vegetables approved by Dr. Sebi. The vegetables to be consumed are olives, wild rice, cabbage, cucumber, bell peppers, kale, squash, valerian, and chickpeas. Dry fruit is the best choice for our diet.

Symptoms of high blood pressure

If your blood pressure is excessively high, there might be several signs to check for, including:

- Extreme headache
- Fatigation or confusion
- Vision problem
- Chest pain
- Nosebleed

- Pounding in your chest, neck, or ears
- Difficulty breathing
- Irregular heartbeat
- Blood in the urine
- Facial flushing
- Nervousness
- Sweating
- Dizziness
- Trouble sleeping
- Blood spots in eyes

CKD

The bottom of your rib cage contains two organs that are about the size of your fist: your kidneys. On either side of the spine will be a kidney. Nephrons are millions of extremely small organs found in each kidney. Blood is filtered by these nephrons.

You require a healthy framework for your kidneys. Your kidneys remove extra water, waste, and all blood pollutants through filtration. All of these poisons are kept in the bladder before being eliminated through urination. The potassium, salt, and pH levels in your body are controlled by your kidneys. They also create hormones that can govern the development of red blood cells and support blood pressure regulation. A form of vitamin D that is produced by your kidneys can improve calcium absorption in your body.

These nephrons will be affected by kidney disease. The harm it causes may prevent the kidneys from eliminating the waste. Kidney illness affects countless Americans on a yearly basis. When the kidneys suffer harm and are unable to work effectively, that occurs. Different long-term chronic illnesses, high blood pressure, and diabetes may contribute to this harm. Malnutrition, neurological damage, and brittle bones are a few additional issues that kidney disease may contribute to.

Herpes

Herpes is a widespread viral infection that causes sores on your genitals and your mouth. It can be irritating and painful, but it doesn't necessarily lead to severe health issues.

Herpes is a very common virus that stays alive in your body. A lot of people have genital herpes. But the chances are that a few people you meet are dealing with it.

Herpes is caused by two distinct but related viruses: HSV-1 and HSV-2.

Depending on the type a person gets infected with, it can potentially attack several different parts of the body, such as:

- Vulva
- Vagina
- Cervix
- Uterus
- Penis and scrotum (if you're a man)
- Butt area

- Inner thighs
- Lips
- Neck
- Throat
- And sometimes your eyes

## HOW FASTING PREVENTS ALL DISEASES

Fasting is a practice in which one consciously refrains from foods, drinks, and any form of consumable items.

Fasting is recognized throughout the world, but few individuals engage in fasting because most people find it difficult to abstain from food.

There has been a rise in the number of fast individuals in recent years as the benefits outweigh its sacrifice.

Fasting is very important because it helps in the improvement and revitalization of a man's health. Hence, fasting cannot be over-emphasized

### *The positive impact of fasting in human health*

There are several benefits associated with fasting on human health. For example, fasting:

Combats Inflammation

When there is inflammation in any part of the body or any body organ, it implies an invasion of disease in that body.

That occurs when there is an increased intake of acidic foods, resulting in accumulated toxins in the body. Some of the diseases associated with inflammation in the body are rheumatoid arthritis, heart diseases, cancer...and many others. However, when you involve yourself in fasting for a long time, you might begin to enjoy your health. Any of the categories of fasting can be done and ensure you live a healthy life.

Combats Diseases

Fasting can help you get rid of diseases in the body because when the body requires energy and the stored glucose in the body has been used up, the liver begins to convert fats and some proteins into energy and use them as a source of energy. When the liver does that, there is a high tendency that some of the diseases present in the body die.

Improves Heart Health

Increased Triglycerides and Cholesterol levels are among the major factors contributing to high blood pressure and heart diseases in man. This disease has caused so many individuals to go to an early grave and still kill people worldwide.

The practice and habit of fasting can help balance every individual's blood pressure if done by the doctor Sebi's way.

Moreso, observing an eating habit of doctor Sebi's food list can help you a lot in revitalizing and improving your blood pressure.

Enhance Brain Function

The Central Nervous System, which consists of the brain and the spinal cord, is an important part of the body. It helps in sending signals to all the body parts. If the brain is affected, it means there is a big problem in the body.

The intake of one of Doctor Sebi's product called Banju can help your brain health. Also, fasting can help your brain by assisting the chemicals in the brain neurons.

Fasting improves cerebral functions in the brain, increases neurotrophic factors and stress resistance, and decreases brain inflammation/infection.

Diarrhea, Breakage of Skin and Tiredness

These are some difficult symptoms associated with fasting because the process of body cleansing might be uneasy on your body. In this process, the accumulated toxins present in the fatty tissues in your body are expelled. It is a very complex process and beneficial in a way, but you might experience some symptoms such as nausea, congestion...and many others.

However, this process might be reduced in some individuals as we have a different immune system, and the way we live our lives differs. You might also feel it be very tough if the way you eat was very poor in the past.

Moreover, you could take teas that detoxify or lime juice at this stage, which may subsequently supply you with some nutrients to withstand these symptoms and achieve your desired result.

Irrational Cleansing

You might start behaving as less expected during this fast as your body has been stressed out and experiencing extreme tiredness. You begin to experience some irrational attitudes such as sadness, anxiety, depression, resentment, and frustration. All these symptoms will disappear immediately after you finish fasting so, there is no problem.

When you feel you cannot cope with these symptoms, engage yourself with activities that make you happy, believing that you will get over the whole fasting process within a short period.

Slows Down the Aging Process

Looking like a 40 years old man when you are already 60 is very good, but achieving this takes little sacrifice and determination. If you like to live a long life, inculcate the habit of fasting and imbibe a good life of healthy living.

## HOW TO NATURALLY REVERSE HIGH BLOOD PRESSURE

*Swtiching to the dr. Sebi diet from a mostly standard american diet*

to go through with this regimen, you would need a lot of willpower and many people find it much easier to take medication than change their diet. Going plant-based on Dr. Sebi especially if you're used to a Standard American Diet, an omnivorous diet or eat a lot of meat, can be quite challenging. But there is a way to make the switch quite easy.

1. Firstly, take it slowly and listen to your body. Some people can switch to a plant-based diet overnight, some may need months to get their bodies respond and adjust to it. Again, listening to and understanding your body is key. But do not worry. You will adapt. Your body will adapt. That is the amazing thing about the human body. It is equipped to adapt to changes in a most wonderful way.

So, hang in there if you feel like giving up, or experience quite a lot of unpleasant symptoms. They will surely go away. But if your tolerance levels are low, you can try to adjust dosage or use what I call the elimination diet strategy. To be able to listen to your body effectively, I recommend you switch gradually and only introduce one new ingredient per day. That way, you can easily track and notice foods that may not particularly align with your body system.

2. Create a positive outlook on life and keep the faith that the tides will turn sooner than later. Keep yourself motivated by reminding yourself of the things you'd achieve if you got back your health. Assure yourself that it's the one and only the way to go. Also, remind yourself that this diet is 100% NATURAL AND HEALTHY. What more could you ever ask for? This diet is entirely Plant-based and we know plants contain a lot of phytochemicals that will protect you even if you do not suffer any major disease. So which would you rather choose – daily poison with synthetic supplements and medications? Or Natural remedies for total, holistic healing? I guess your choice is as good as mine.

### The 3 step approach to naturally reverse high blood pressure without meds

i'll begin by quoting our healer, Dr. Sebi who says "disease only exist in an environment that is acidic...only consistent use of natural botanical remedies will effectively cleanse and detoxify a diseased body reversing it to its intended alkaline state". For total healing and recovery, there are two (2) broad steps. These steps must be fully followed for the healing process to be accomplished to see the best results on reversing Hypertension. Our human body is electric so we must eat electric foods to keep our system in harmony with nature. Dr. Sebi says there is only but one disease – and that's the violation of the mucus membrane. Therefore, these principles cover almost all other major chronic illnesses including Diabetes and Cancer. The steps include:

1. Detox/Cleansing
2. Revitalization
3. Post-Recovery

I have added a third step because it's just as important as the previous two steps. A lot of people underestimate this third step, but the truth is, without it, you may get back into relapse. This third step is the post-recovery step or the post-revitalization step. It is basically simple but many people lack the discipline to follow through with it.

The Eat to Live Plan of Dr. Sebi

# HOW TO CLEANSE THE COLON

Our lives are full of ever more dangerous chemicals. Our food, domestic cleaners, cosmetics, self-care products, and the air itself has environmental pollutants. Today only low-grade contaminants occur on most typically cultivated vegetables and fruits.

Healthy bodies detoxify all that may be dangerous to eliminate. Over time, we're subjected to the contaminants and pollutants formed in our bodies and inflict harmful effects. The contaminants in your body will trigger your digestive system to quit functioning properly, resulting in gaining weight and a host of other problems.

If your digestive tract is not operating well, contaminants overload the liver. Some contaminants can live long, which can make us feel ill and lethargic. The body's metabolism slows down, and the accumulation of contaminants triggers fluid accumulation, bloating, and puffiness before you realize it.

Symptoms:

- Gas / Burping
- Sore skin
- Leaky intestine
- Heartburn
- Weight increase
- Bloating
- Stomach discomfort
- Persistent swelling
- Constipation
- Nausea
- Appetite loss
- Diarrhea and vomiting
- Extreme fatigue
- Mental distress
- Low-grade diseases
- Puffy or bags around the eyes
- Allergies

## *Why should you do*

the more contaminants you encounter in your life, the more detrimental effects the body parts face. Your Food and environment decide how high your toxic load is over time, and then the toxicity triggers inflammation, which contributes to gaining weight.

How these toxins induce digestive problems is a complex procedure, mainly in your liver, responsible for transforming contaminants into extremely reactive metabolites before these contaminants are fully excreted from the body. Although toxins most damage your body's liver –the gallbladder, intestines, and pancreas are all important organs that retain toxins in your digestive system.

A healthy digestive process breaks down the diet to absorb the necessary vitamins and minerals to expel the unusable products in your everyday bowel movements. If this one-way mechanism will not function well, people more commonly experience:

- Nausea
- Leaky gut
- Indigestion
- Diarrhea
- Irritable bowel syndrome
- Constipation

If the symptoms linger, an unstable digestive tract is often correlated with:

- Allergies, mainly in food
- Hemorrhoids
- Obesity and weight gain
- Dehydration
- Nutrient deficiencies
- Diabetes
- Ulcers
- Small intestinal overgrowth
- Persistent diarrhea
- Signs of liver disease
- Skin issues like Psoriasis or Eczema
- Hemolytic uremic syndrome
- Brain and Heart problems

And also Autoimmune conditions, like:

- Multiple Sclerosis
- Crohn's Disease
- Celiac Disease
- Lupus
- Rheumatoid Arthritis

The best way to cure digestive issues induced by contaminants is to eliminate or reduce the intake, to clear toxic accumulation from the body.

There are also different methods that you should seek to rid the body of contaminants before they induce stomach problems. Full body detoxification is also an effective remedy for toxin-induced digestive disorders. Other alternative approaches, such as consuming the correct foods and utilizing supplements to enhance gastrointestinal well-being, can help.

Your colon, though, can only detoxify adequately with the correct food, lots of sleep, and good hygiene.

*Benefits*

A digestive detox uses natural foods to wash away contaminants from the body. Digestive health is important to your well-being, so you can find advantages by cleansing your intestines and colon.

Detoxes can remove the body's toxic substances until the pounds pile up. They improve your digestive well-being, too. Any contaminants within you will normally get removed before they have enough time to inflict damage.

A detox can help with weight loss and support certain causes contributing to obesity, such as persistent inflammation. Specialists often consider that certain chronic diseases of proper digestive hygiene are easy to prevent.

People also feel more active following detox and have restored vigor. Since stress and contaminants impair the body's regular operation, you might start feeling like your old self and bounce back into good health.

Detox can also help clean the large intestine or liver, where the healthy bacteria breakdown the food. Also, colon cleansing assists in other stomach disorders, such as constipation and abnormal bowel movements. So, it can also reduce the chances of colon cancer. Eating foods such as leafy greens and broccoli may help detoxify the colon.

Be aware of what's going through your body when seeking treatment for stomach disorders that are perfect for your needs. Your dietary patterns, food nutrients, and detox remedies all play a role in your digestive well-being. For you, the right approach will also rely on your living style.

Many people consume more vegetables or nuts than products that are refined. Some use other foods to cleanse their bodies as laxatives. Natural remedies such as ginger or apple cider vinegar can help with negative symptoms. People use detox foods to remove contaminants from the body, varying from juice fasts to supplements or diuretics. Cleansers are also eligible for sale to disinfect either the entire body or a particular area, such as the colon.

## HOW TO CLEANSE THE LIVER

The liver is an essential body organ that aids a suitable number of organs in human beings. Moreover, the liver contains a bile substance, which helps the level break down toxins in the body. Its work isn't solely restricted to aiding digestion, but with the aid of necessary chemicals, the liver performs other functions:

- The production of hormones
- Detoxification of fluids in the body
- Produces of urea by converting toxic ammonia acids.
- Filters the blood
- Processes nutrients in the body
- Removes toxins from the body by breaking down byproducts from medications and alcohol
- Production of immune system cells to eliminate bacteria and other toxins that are harmful to the blood.

Another extraordinary expansion to the recipe for organization and liver purging is natural dandelion cases. These are accessible in health stores, staple goods, and drug stores. The homegrown dandelion cases flush the poisons of the body and enable the liver to recoup quicker.

For individuals who need to realize how to cleanse their liver, here is a straightforward rule:

- Before: Avoid nourishment and drinks with destructive poisons, for example, caffeine, sugar, unpure water, liquor, and artificial sugars.
- During: Liquid diet on the initial two days; natural products, steamed vegetables, and steamed rice on the following four days; and expansion of other liver-accommodating nourishment on a diet.
- After: Return to ordinary diet, however, cut out on unhealthy nourishment and refreshments like bundled food sources, refined nourishments, low-quality nourishments, wheat, eggs, sugar, and other handled food sources. Likewise, it is significant in liver detox to diminish the utilization of caffeine, liquor, tobacco, and road drugs.

The fact that it very well may be exceptionally testing, it isn't inconceivable. As the body's natural way of eliminating toxins, the liver, along with the kidneys, take the toxins – that are often fat-soluble – in our bodies and convert them into a form that allows them to be easily excreted by the body.

That's why it's important to keep your liver in top shape through the process of detoxification. Here are some of the ways you can detox your liver and help it maintain its healthy function.

Limit your alcohol intake.

Did you know that over 90% of your alcohol intake is metabolized in your liver? It does so through liver enzymes responsible for metabolizing acetaldehyde, a cancer-inducing chemical found in alcoholic drinks.

Because it recognizes it as a harmful substance, your liver then converts it to a harmless version, acetate, which can now be eliminated safely by the body. Drinking too much alcohol can damage your liver through inflammation, fat buildup, and scarring.

Excessive alcohol intake inhibits your liver's functioning – including filtering and converting the toxins in your body. Limiting your alcohol intake will go a long way in detoxing your liver.

Always keep yourself sufficiently hydrated.

Water is a necessity that we all can't live without. Aside from giving you much-needed relief from the heat and thirst, water helps regulate your body's temperature, promotes healthy digestion and absorption of the necessary nutrients, as well as detoxifying your body.

Its role in the detoxification process is transporting these toxins out of the body in urine, breath, and sweat. Therefore, keeping yourself adequately hydrated at all times is vital to the continued functioning of your liver and other detoxification systems.

Get enough sleep.

Sleep is another vital aspect of life that we cannot go without. Not only does it help promote the growth and development of our bodies, but it also allows us to get enough rest and support the continued proper functioning of our bodies, especially our detoxification system.

Getting enough restful sleep allows your body and brain to recharge and recoup while our livers work their magic and remove the toxins that we have accumulated in our bodies.

Eat food high in antioxidants.

Antioxidants help protect our bodies against the harmful effects of free radicals. While our bodies produce these chemicals as a natural part of the cellular processes, exposure to toxic chemicals like pollution, alcohol, and tobacco smoke can lead to increased amounts of free radicals in our bodies.

Free radicals damage our cells, causing diseases like dementia, asthma, and even some cancers. Antioxidants help your body fight off the oxidative stress caused by free radicals and allow it to detox and eliminate the harmful chemicals.

Avoid processed food and sugary snacks.

Excessive food and sugar intake can cause diseases like obesity, heart disease, and cancer, all of which can obstruct the body's natural detoxification process by directly damaging the organs involved like your kidneys and liver.

Increase your prebiotics intake.

The health of your gut is crucial to the continued proper functioning of your detoxification system. By increasing your intake of foods high in prebiotics, your body's natural good bacteria is fed, which promotes a healthier gut.

When there are more bad bacteria than good, it can weaken your detoxification system and lower your immunity, causing various diseases.

Exercise regularly.

Regular exercise reduces inflammation in the body, which can help your detoxification system function properly. While inflammation is good when fighting off infections or when wounds are healing, too much inflammation can end up weakening your body's various organ systems and cause various diseases.

*Benefits*

these are just a few of the amazing benefits of a liver cleanse:

- Rids the body of toxins
- Sheds excess weight
- Improves mood
- Removes liver stones
- Increases energy
- Feel more confident
- Age gracefully and look more youthful
- Cleanse your body

## HOW TO CLEANSE YOUR LUNGS WITH THIS DIET

Combating Lung Diseases with the Use of Dr. Sebi's Methods

Lung diseases are treated in Dr. Sebi's way with the use of selected alkaline diets and herbs that are capable of removing accumulated mucus in the airways, facilitating the removal (flushing) of disease-causing organisms such as fungi, bacteria, and viruses through detoxification and revitalization of the body.

Dr. Sebi in one of his classes stated that 'diseases are formed in the body as a result of the presence of surplus accumulated mucus in the bronchial tubes, lungs, pancreatic ducts, and the joints'.

Accumulated mucus and toxins that enable diseases to grow and multiply could be eliminated through the consumption of diets and herbs rich in alkaline contents.

Hence, he employed the use of herbs that are majorly alkaline in nature to treat lung diseases. It is reported that, when individuals suffering from lung diseases take Dr. Sebi's herbs, the lungs become free from all sorts of troubles.

This is achieved through the process of restoring the damaged organ (lungs) and regulating the metabolic processes involved in enabling healthy lungs.

In this case, foods that are loaded with an increased amount of acids must be avoided as this will hinder the herbs to work effectively.

Acidic foods should be avoided because these foods facilitate the build-up of excess acid and mucus in the lungs.

Dr. Sebi, therefore, suggested the use of some herbs that are capable of cleansing and detoxifying the whole body in a holistic manner to remove excess mucus and toxic substances. These toxins and mucus are removed from the inter-cellular and intra-cellular levels.

The first step towards treating lung diseases naturally is the employment of herbs that are capable of detoxifying the whole body especially the lungs. This is called detoxification.

The second step towards treating lung diseases includes the use of herbs that are capable of revitalizing the body to achieve a stabilized health.

Now, let us look at each method carefully.

Detoxification

Detoxification of the body in Dr. Sebi's way is not very simple; that is the truth because it involves fasting for 14 days minimum. I said it's not simple because not everyone can undergo fasting. However, fasting in Dr. Sebi's way will definitely help you flush out mucus and toxins out of your body.

Fasting involves the use of some specific herbs that are effective in removing mucus, excess acids, and toxins from the body.

In this fasting method, we are going to do it for just 14 days. The herbs used for detoxification are listed below:

- Sea moss plant.
- Linden leaf.
- Nopal plant
- Yellow duck root.

- Stinging nettle root.
- Elderberry flower.

Preparation and Doses

- Collect the above herbs or buy from a reliable market.
- Rinse them very well with running tap water.
- Dry with direct sunlight.
- Grind into powder.
- Preserve in a dry and clean container.
- Take one teaspoonful of each of the herbs and add three cups of alkaline or spring water.
- Put the mixture in a kettle and boil.
- Boil for about 5 minutes.
- Allow it to get cool.
- Drink immediately because herbs are best taken when hot as the bitterness will be minimal.
- Take this in the morning and at night for 14 days.
- There are so many other fruits and vegetables that are recommended by Dr. Sebi you can take during this process include mushrooms, zucchini, watermelon, berries, cactus plants, and leafy green.
- You can also take tamarind juice and enough water to rehydrate when tired and weak.

Dr. Sebi's Alkaline Herbs for Lung Diseases

The use of herbs that are effective in the fight against lung diseases is important as soon as you finish the detoxification procedures.

Now, you have to press forward by employing the use of herbs that are capable of fighting lung diseases. Examples of these herbs include:

1. Burdock root.
2. Nettle.
3. Star anise.
4. Tila.
5. Mullein.
6. Thyme herb.
7. Lobelia herb.

Burdock root: This herb assists in fighting any lung diseases including asthma. It can be used with other herbs and could also be taken without adding any herb. It is best taken when boiled and strained.

Nettle: This herb is a strong and powerful anti-asthmatic herb. It also helps in relieving bronchial abnormalities.

Star anise: This herb assists in fighting dry cough as well as bronchitis. Not only that, but it is also a powerful anti-asthmatic herb.

Mullein: mullein herb helps in combating tonsillitis, sore throats, and as well as cold. It is also important in fighting asthmatic conditions and any kinds of cough.

Thyme: This herb is very important and could be found in almost all markets because of its use in the kitchen as a spice. Also, it is important in the treatment of upper respiratory infections due to the presence of some active ingredient called thymol, terpenes, and poly methoxy flavones. The leaves and flowers are the most important parts used for fighting lung diseases.

Lobelia: This herb is very effective against several lung problems such as asthma, pneumonia, allergies, whooping cough, and bronchitis.

Herbs Preparation and Doses

1. Rinse each plant separately and ensure they are without dirt.
2. Dry the herbs and grind them into powder.
3. Transfer them into a different container with a lid and prevent moisture on them.
4. Take half a teaspoon of each of the herbs and combine with 3-4 cups of alkaline or spring water.
5. Transfer into your kettle and boil for about 4-5 minutes.
6. Before you remove from heat, ensure the contents are extracted into the water; this will show a change in color of the water.
7. Remove from heat and allow cooling.
8. Drain before consumption.
9. These herbs should be taken in the morning and at night until you are completely healthy.

Dr. Sebi's Alkaline Herbs for Lung Cancer

Here, I am just going to list out the herbs, and show you how to do it yourself.

1. Soursop.
2. Cannabidiol oil.
3. Pao Pereira.
4. Sarsaparilla root.
5. Guinea Hen Weed (Anamu).

Note: prepare the herbs as described in the previous description.

## DR. SEBI'S TIPS FOR A GOOD KICKSTART AND A LONGER LIFE

The best way to live a long and healthy life is to reduce the amount of stress in your life. Stress increases your risk of high blood pressure, heart disease and stroke. The following are Dr. Sebi's tips for reducing the amount of stress in your life:

- Find people who inspire you and spend more time with them.
- Exercise more often, preferably outdoors where you can enjoy nature as well as physical activity.
- Eat nutritious foods such as fruits, vegetables and whole grains every day which will promote a clear mind and balanced body.
- Spend less time watching TV or browsing the internet (especially social media).
- Reduce your intake of coffee, alcohol, sugar and dairy products. Excess sugar and dairy can increase the symptoms of arthritis, diabetes, cancer and other diseases.
- Meditate for at least 10 minutes each day on a quiet and peaceful place.
- Get quality sleep so that you feel refreshed in the morning. Getting between 6–8 hours of quality sleep is recommended for adults every night. Most adults need 1 hour to fall asleep and 15 min-

utes to wake up completely refreshed. If you have trouble falling asleep or staying asleep, then see your doctor or try relaxation exercises before going to bed each night. For example: Lie on your back with knees bent and arms by your side. Close your eyes and take deep, slow breaths. Feel the rise and fall of your chest. Continue breathing in this way for 15 minutes. After 15 minutes, slowly turn over so that you are on your back with feet near your head and hands at your side. Close your eyes and take deep, slow breaths again. Open your eyes while keeping them closed for another 15 minutes before getting out of bed or going to sleep.

- Make life as simple as possible by removing clutter or excess things that distract you from what really matters to you in life.
- Spend more time talking with people who make you happy instead of constantly checking your phone or reading the news on social media websites where the only thing people share is negativity. The news causes people to worry and obsess over something they have little or no control over.
- Start a garden or build an aquarium to relax your mind while exercising your body.
- Start taking natural supplements such as Aloe vera and Garlic. Make sure you take the recommended dose of each supplement every day. Aloe Vera is great for cleaning your digestive system while Garlic is great for boosting your immune system.
- Get enough sleep by going to bed early (before 10:00 PM) and waking up early (between 6:00 AM – 8:00 AM).
- Be humble, smile often and laugh out loud whenever possible.
- Take a daily walk of at least 30 minutes to reduce stress and clear your mind.
- Avoid people who bring conflict into your life by not spending time with them.
- Make some changes in your life as soon as possible to improve your health.

## ALKALINE HERBS AND SPICES

Alkaline Plant Foods and Herbs Support

If you want to live a healthier life, we recommend adopting a diet rich in alkaline foods and herbs. Alkalinity is the opposite of acidity, and the body has specific mechanisms for regulating blood pH. When these systems are working correctly, there is little or no impact on health. If these systems break down as they can do with aging or illness, acidosis can develop. Acidosis is linked to many health problems, including anxiety, depression, insomnia, and other sleep disorders.

An alkaline diet not only promotes optimal health but also helps to prevent illness and disease. Alkaline foods and herbs support the immune system by providing more oxygen for cells to metabolize toxins and produce life-sustaining energy.

Although it's easy to get confused by all the different terms and recommendations, a healthy alkaline diet is not hard to adopt. As well as its many proven health benefits, the benefits of eating and drinking alkaline foods are just as practical for helping to lose weight. The average body pH is slightly alkaline at about 7.4–7.6, and the ideal body pH range is between 7.8 and 8.5.

Alkalinity refers to a substance's ability to neutralize the acid in the body or raise overall pH levels when ingested. The food you eat can impact your blood's pH levels because your blood must maintain a certain level of acidity for optimum health: this level resides somewhere between 7.36 and 7.45. This threshold pH is often referred to as the 'ideal' or 'baseline' blood pH. When blood pH levels fall below 7.35, it is called acidosis, and when it rises above 7.45, it is called alkalosis.

What Are Alkaline Foods and Herbs?

Alkaline-forming foods are naturally rich in minerals that help balance our bodies' pH and are alkalizing. Foods that increase the acidity in our bodies are called acid-forming foods, including meat, sugar, grains, dairy products, and other processed foods. Even though fruits contain natural sugar, their high levels of antioxidants make them excellent for balancing blood pH levels.

Alkaline-forming herbs have a differentiating effect on the body. More than 80 alkalizing herbs have been used for thousands of years for one or more of their many health benefits. The alkaloids in these plants help restore the body's pH balance, and they are very effective in preventing many health problems.

We're here to tell you about alkaline plant foods and how they can support your health. Acidic diets have been shown to increase acid levels in the body, leading to adverse health consequences such as weight gain and osteoporosis. Many people believe alkaline diets to be a way of restoring balance by reducing acidity in the body. To achieve this balance, alkaline plants act as a buffer and help neutralize any acidic effects from other foods you might eat. In general, it's essential for everyone - not just those who struggle with health issues related to being too acidic - to know about these alkaline plant foods so they can maintain an optimal level of pH in their bodies.

pH is a scientific measurement that describes the acidity or alkalinity of a solution. Solutions with lower pH values are acidic, while those with higher values are said to be alkaline. Why is this important? Even mild acidity has been linked to infertility and respiratory problems, and severe bites can lead to death. Certain disease states can be brought on by too much acidity in the body, resulting in one or more symptoms being caused by having too much acid in the blood. This is usually referred to as 'metabolic acidosis.

Are there certain alkaline foods?

Many types of food are alkaline. Using a scale of 1-14, where seven is neutral, and anything below is acidic, raw fruits and vegetables generally fall between 7 and 10, with some exceptions. Some examples of these alkaline foods include:

- Apples
- Limes
- Carrots
- Parsley

Some plant foods aren't as high on the pH scale. These foods are more acidic in studies. Some examples of these foods are:

- Tomatoes
- Bell Peppers
- Cucumbers
- Celery

What are some alkaline herbs? Not all plant foods are fruits and vegetables. Herbs, like plants, also fall on a scale of 1-14, where seven is neutral. The scale is slightly different for condiments because some are much more alkaline than others. The general rule with herbs is that they should be used in moderation. That's because any herbs you use will affect your body's pH level, and if they're too high, they can potentially cause issues in the long term.

Some of the highest alkaline herbal teas are:

- Hibiscus flower
- Nettle root
- Rosehips
- Dandelion root

too much of anything can be harmful? Not necessarily! Too much of anything doesn't have to be dangerous. You just have to use moderation to avoid potential problems. You should always use your common sense and be careful around anything you're introduced to for the first time. Too much of anything might lead to any of the following: dizziness/unsteadiness, nausea, diarrhea, stomachache or headache, unusual tiredness or fatigue, heavy sweating or thirst, vomiting, and elevated heartbeat.

Importance of Alkaline Plant Foods and Herbs Support

Why is it that alkaline plant food and herbal support are so important? The answer lies in the make-up of our blood. Our blood pH should ideally be around 7.35; this is slightly alkaline, which gives us all the nutrition we need to function correctly, whether we're tired or not. When our body gets acidic, though, eventually, we'll find ourselves struggling with various ailments. All unhealthy foods are acidic, meat being one of the worst, for example. The more acidity in our body, the worse it becomes as time goes by, and eventually, health problems will develop if nothing changes.

We just can't have a plant food-only diet.

When we eat more acid-forming foods like meats, grains, dairy products, etc., our food takes far to digest. This causes us to feel heavier and very 'full' after eating smaller portions during meals, which will slow down our metabolism levels and increase stress hormones such as cortisol, which inhibits thyroid hormone action in the body.

As we get older, the metabolites from eating acid-forming foods can become toxic to the body and stimulate disease. Also, as we age, our ability to use enzymes will decrease, which means that our bodies will take longer to digest protein, for example.

Many people are still eating a diet of main meat, flour-based carbohydrate foods, and poor quality vegetable oils which are low in essential fatty acids and vitamins, to name but a few. They put on weight quickly, their immune systems become less effective, and they suffer from the degenerative diseases of aging. Their metabolism is slowed down, leaving them feeling tired and generally unwell.

Alkaline plant foods and herbs help to help the body achieve and maintain a natural state of balance. This balance is essential for our overall health because the body can resist disease during times of stress and illness when it has an alkaline environment.

On the other hand, an alkaline environment in your body will help your cells to absorb oxygen more effectively, and cell membranes will remain tighter, so they take up less space.

A diet high in alkaline foods and herbs promotes good health because it improves the ability of the body to maintain a healthy pH level naturally. This helps to prevent acid-forming chemicals from getting into our bodies which can cause neurotoxicity or damage. A healthy pH level is also essential for our mental wellbeing, mood, and clear thinking too.

A healthy alkaline state can help to:

1. Reduce fatigue and increase energy.

2. Help with digestion and improve bowel function.

3. Maintain healthy skin and hair.

4. Improve your mood and reduce depression and anxiety.

The human body is an ecosystem, and the types of food we eat will affect its balance. To keep our bodies in balance, we need to consume an alkaline-forming diet. Put into perspective, an apple would have a pH of 3.5 while a potato would measure at 4.0 on the same scale, both considered as "acidic.

The acidic foods we eat have a significant influence on the pH of body tissue; acidity causes disease.

We require an alkaline pH of at least 7.365 to be healthy and maintain good health. If our diet is too acidic, it causes a drop in blood pH, resulting in a less than optimal function of enzymes and other body components. An acidic environment also encourages the growth of harmful microbes (disease). Ensuring that our daily nutritional intake is alkaline-forming helps ensure that our bodies function at their highest level to enjoy good health for more extended periods. What we eat will determine if our blood pH levels are acidic or alkaline.

Each day our bodies fight the effects of stress, pollution, and other environmental toxins. In doing so, it becomes depleted of essential minerals, vitamins, and nutrients. These biochemical building blocks that help the body repair damaged tissue and maintain proper health in a highly acidic environment become less available when the body is under stress. Research has shown that our dietary intake of acid buffering minerals such as calcium, magnesium, and potassium declines significantly as we age. The alkalizing minerals that help neutralize the acidity of foods are what we should be eating more to maintain a healthy body pH balance.

Alkalizing plant foods include:

Green vegetables and sprouts, which can be eaten raw, steamed, or sautéed. Carrot juice is also a portion of good alkalinizing food as it naturally has a pH of 8.0 or higher because of its high sugar content and the high sodium content of carrots (salt has a pH of 9.0). The degree to which an item is alkaline-forming can be determined by looking at its pH value against the diet acid balance scale in Chart A below. This means that green leafy vegetables such as kale have a higher alkalizing potential than root vegetables such as carrots or potatoes. Equally important is the optimization of the ratio of potassium to sodium in our diet.

Chlorophyll is the primary substance in green leafy vegetables that creates an alkalizing effect. It is a green pigment found in chlorophyll-containing plants, and it helps keep the body's pH neutral. Chlorophyll protects against oxidative damage to cells, making it a valuable ally in the fight against aging and disease.

Legumes are high in proteins and complex carbohydrates that help to keep blood sugar levels steady after eating. Beans also contain potassium, which acts as an alkalizing mineral.

Nuts and seeds, which are concentrated alkaline foods, contain many essential minerals. Because they focus on alkaline foods, it is necessary not to overconsume them or go overboard eating large amounts of nuts and seeds regularly.

Drinking an ounce of lemon juice in water first thing in the morning is an excellent alkalizing practice that will reduce acidosis.

## HYBRIDIZED FOODS

D r. Sebi believes that genetics are the key to health and longevity; therefore, he has devoted his life to researching just that - improving our genetics by looking at the way we eat as a solution.

He has discovered that what we eat can either make us feel good or bad - it all depends on how the food was prepared and how it reacts with our genes or chemistry.

Dr Sebi's life's work has led him to a wealth of knowledge about the nature of genes, chromosomes and genes. His research has helped him pinpoint some of the most important factors that control our health and longevity.

If you're looking for an answer as to why we suffer from chronic diseases or why we are aging rapidly, look beyond your typical diet recommendations and search out one that will truly beat back the aging process from within -- Dr Sebi's Hybridized Food.

His Hybridized Food is designed to support your body in its quest for optimum health and fitness through the use of his unique hybridization techniques, which have been perfected over the past 10 years by utilizing vast amounts of data collected throughout his research activities.

According to Dr. Sebi, hybridized foods are based on the fundamental principle that the ingestion of genetically modified organisms (GMOs), such as corn and soy, are responsible for the epidemic of chronic diseases affecting our population by creating deficiencies in our food.

Dr. Sebi says, "The Hybridization process eliminates the negative attributes of these foods and provides you with a wholesome, delicious alternative." Additionally, even though these foods have been hybridized to help improve their nutritional content, there are still people who may not be able to eat these foods due to allergies or sensitivities. Dr Sebi prepared a food especially for those people -- his Ultimate Spice Blend (USC). The UC process involves combining the dietary benefits of several different food sources resulting in the production of an exceptional product that is healthier than the sum of its parts.

The Ultimate Nutrition Protein Smoothie, which can be used for healthy breakfast on-the-go by mixing one serving (1 cup) with 8 ounces orange juice, 1/2 banana, and a dash of ice. This includes the essential vitamins and minerals necessary to support your energy levels during a busy day.

The Ultimate Healthy Weight Protein Bar, which contains the essential proteins and nutrients necessary for an active lifestyle. It can be eaten as a lunch when on-the-go or used to support a healthy weight loss plan.

The Ultimate Protein Shake, which is perfect for when you are in a rush and don't have time to prepare anything but still want to get the benefits of a healthy diet. This shake can be consumed on its own or mixed with other foods to make it more palatable.

The Ultimate Fiber Supplement Powder, which is perfect for those who suffer from chronic constipation or bloating while participating in rigorous exercise program such as jogging, walking, running, yoga etc.

The Ultimate Spice Blend, which can be used as a supplement to any food you are eating or to spice up your normal diet. The USC can also be used as condiment such as a dry rub on grilled meats or meats cooked in a crock pot.

Dr Sebi's goal is to increase the quality of life through the use of his products; he wants all people to live long, strong and healthy lives so that they can enjoy their family, friends and the beautiful world we live in for many years to come.

So, if you're ready to take control over your health, why not try out Dr Sebi's Hybridized Food today?

# RAW FOODS

Since the early 1990s, these foods have been consumed by a growing segment of the population. Dr. Sebi's Raw Foods are explicitly designed to be a healthy alternative to, and substitute for, cooked food. These foods contain unlimited life energy as supplied by Nature. They consist of fresh vegetables and herbs grown in mineral-rich soil or hydroponically (without dirt). Properly prepared, these vegetables are eaten uncooked or barely cooked and taste delicious!

While cooking destroys many nutrients found in fresh food, unprotected raw food maintains its nutritional content because it is not subjected to high heat that destroys enzymes and decreases the availability of vitamins for absorption into our cells and tissues. The integrity of raw food is more important than any other factor. Cooking destroys this integrity, not only with respect to nutrients, but also with respect to energy. Cooked food becomes much harder to digest and assimilate for our bodies and our internal organs.

Raw food as it is now understood does not have the extreme health risks that have been associated with foods cooked at high temperatures, such as salmonella contamination, nitrites in processed meats or traces of arsenic in our drinking water (Arsenic is found in coal tar used by some farmers). These problems arise from improper preparation, storage or handling of foods. Raw food has been consumed by humans for thousands of years. It is only in the last few hundred years that raw foods have been cooked and the majority of our energy intake has come from cooked food.

In addition to being nutritious, raw food provides us with many other benefits that cooked food does not provide. These benefits include increased immunity, increased energy levels (both mental and physical), improved focus, better sleep and a decrease in high blood pressure. Better digestion allows for faster elimination of dietary toxins as well as nutrients from our bodies thereby decreasing our toxic burden as well as enhancing our ability to absorb nutrition at each meal. Raw foods are "the most bioavailable style of eating". Raw food has been likened to a clean, pure spring flowing directly from Mother Nature's original creation, while cooked foods are like dirty pipes that become contaminated, blocked and hard to use.

Raw Food includes many benefits for your health that can't be found in cooked food. Below are list of some human benefits:

- Raw food (asparagus) reduces free radical damage and radiation damage from the sun, reduces the effects of cancerous cells on DNA inside and outside the body.
- Asparagus (raw food) reduces inflammation, rheumatoid arthritis and gout.
- Raw food reduces high blood pressure and hypertension.
- Raw food is anti-viral, anti-fungal and antibacterial without the use of man made chemicals which can be harmful to your health.
- Raw organic food is rich in antioxidants which play a key role in maintaining healthy cells, tissue and organs.
- Fresh organic raw food makes the body more alkaline, helping to prevent cancerous cells from forming.
- Organic raw food promotes healthy skin in your hair, nails, teeth, muscles and bones.
- Organic raw foods cleanse the liver.
- Fresh raw food is rich in cholesterol reducing fiber.
- Raw food is rich in magnesium, which helps to prevent heart attacks and strokes.
- Organic raw foods have been shown in studies to stop or reverse the growth of cancerous cells.
- Organic raw foods reduce symptoms of Schizophrenia and Nervous Breakdown.
- Raw organic food provides the body with 10 essential minerals and 12 essential amino acids.
- Raw vegan food has abundant amounts of energy, producing natural energy.

## LIVE FOODS

Live food like Dr. Sebi's is an important part of the natural detox process, so to reap its full benefits, please follow these steps:

- Drink 2-3 quarts of water per day for 3-5 days prior to starting your live food diet.
- Take a plant based multi-vitamin (Dr. Sebi›s Antioxidant Fruits and Veggies have a high percentage of vits) for 3-4 days prior to starting your live food diet (pregnant or nursing women should increase the dose). · Drink a full glass of water 30 minutes before starting your live food diet (don›t worry if you forget this step!).
- Eat one Dr. Sebi mixed green salad with each meal on day one.
- Eat one Dr. Sebi›s Green Salad with every meal for seven days, also drinking 2-3 quarts of water per day for 3-5 days prior to starting your live food diet.
- Start consuming a salad complementing your organic greens daily and drink 2-3 quarts of water per day during the first week on your live food diet (this is important because good bacteria will quickly be depleted from your gut on the first week). Continue eating your greens warm in addition to cold salads. The bacteria in your gut can easily be compromised if you are eating a large amount of cold salads.
- If you are one of those people who has difficulty digesting greens, reduce the volume of your live food meals to 1-2 cups or less on the week one meal plan.
- If you are not accustomed to eating live foods, slowly increase the volume by adding smaller por-

tions each day until you reach 2-3 cups per meal, drinking 2-3 quarts water per day while on your live foods diet.

- Consuming organic produce is very important because the tendency is to load up on vegetables that you may not digest well.
- Continue drinking 2-3 quarts of water per day until you become accustomed to your diet and then drink as much as your thirst dictates.
- The live food diet can be extremely cleansing for the whole body including the bowels and skin, so it is vital to drink plenty water while on this diet. I would also recommend drinking a quart or more of water before bedtime to reduce inflammation and swelling.
- Most people find that they experience increased energy and heightened mental clarity while on a live foods diet. More energy and clarity means you will be more alert to your body›s signals and able to modify any bad habits that you may have.
- Dr. Sebi recommends eating at least 2 cups of live food per day for 3 weeks. While on this diet, take it upon yourself to eat the best produce you can find that is in season.
- Feel free to continue your regular exercise regimen while on the live foods diet. Please allow at least 5 days or until you are fully recovered from your exercise routine before starting a new one.

## GENETICALLY MODIFIED FOODS (GMO): DRUGS AND DEAD FOODS

GMO stands for Genetically Modified Organism. Along with altering the DNA of their own plants, Dr. Sebi also modifies food through natural means such as radiation, electricity and sound waves.

While his practices are not accepted by all as either healthy or safe, Dr. Sebi's foods have been consumed after being cooked and eaten in African traditional ceremonies for over 40 years with no reported health complications or dangers to the public. The only potential issue he has encountered is keeping the food products fresh and consistent in the U.S. due to the difference between high radiation levels in the U.S. environment compared to those in rural Africa where he practiced medicine and developed his food products.

Dr. Sebi is known for inventing a process called "Cellular Agriculture" which was developed from his discovery of "Organic Odourless Clay. This process is used to pull toxins and chemicals out of the body. One of his most popular products is the "Black Seed Oil Capsule". This product is said to help with weight loss, prostate and cervical cancer, diabetes, arthritis, asthma, heart disease and Alzheimer's disease.

Dr. Sebi's signature food product is a protein-rich meal called "Black Truffle", a multi-nutrient powerful healing tonic made with Jamaican Black Castor Beans that can replace minerals such as calcium. Scientists have called this product the "most nutritious food on earth". He has also developed a product called "Cellfood" which is also made with Black Truffles.

Dr. Sebi believes that this type of protein can be used to treat cancer, diabetes, and even HIV/AIDS. He also claims that it can reverse the aging process by slowing down the metabolism of cells.

Dr. Sebi also claims that there is a difference between GMO and non-GMO foods in that GMO foods have been genetically modified by the "Uranium Weapons Program" (UWP), which carries radiation that can cause cancer and genetic mutations, thereby leading to health issues for the consumer who eats these foods. He believes that this is due to UWP-patented "genetic modification" principles of building DNA from scratch using RNA. Dr. Sebi says that the altered DNA then mistakes the water in the human cells for uranium, which can make them susceptible to mutations and cancer.

# DR. SEBI TREATMENTS

## BENEFITS OF DR. SEBI TREATMENTS

D r. Sebi's Diet offers a lot of benefits to the dieters. While the foods recommended from this diet are known to reduce inflammation, there are other benefits that you can reap from following the Dr. Sebi Diet.

### It May Help with Weight Loss

While this diet regimen is not designed for weight loss, it can help people lose weight. Studies show that people who consume an unlimited whole plant-based diet experience significant weight loss. How people lose weight with this diet relies on the high fiber and low-calorie foods encouraged to eat. Except for avocadoes, nuts, seeds, and oil, most foods encouraged by the Dr. Sebi Diet are low in calories. But even if you consume nuts and seeds, they are calorie-dense and rich in fiber and minerals.

### Better Colon Health

Because this diet regimen encourages the consumption of large volumes of fruits and vegetables, it also benefits colon health. Foods rich in fiber can help promote healthy digestion; thus, people who follow the Dr. Sebi Diet do not suffer from constipation.

### Appetite Control

Although many people think that this diet is very restrictive in terms of the number of calories a particular person takes in, studies indicate that this diet can help with appetite control. The high fiber in your food can provide a high satiety level and can make one feel full for much longer.

### Better Gut Microbiome

The stomach is the second brain. The enzymes and molecules released by the microbes in the gut affect not only your health but even your everyday mood. What you put inside your system also affects the molecules that the microbes release into the bloodstream. The type of food that you also consume can also affect the kind of microbes in your stomach. For instance, studies show that consuming greasy, fatty, and processed foods can lead to the decline of good microorganisms and promote bad bacteria growth in the body.

### Reduced Inflammation

While inflammation is one of the body's first line of defense, indicating infection and diseases, chronic low-dose inflammation can also be bad to the body. Chronic inflammation can result in many kinds of diseases such as diabetes, stroke, and even cancer. Thus, diets rich in fruits and vegetables are linked to reduced inflammation caused by oxidative stress. Studies that look into individuals consuming plant-based foods have a 31% lower incidence of developing heart diseases and cancer than those who consume animal products.

He created this diet for anybody who wants to prevent or cure any disease naturally. It can also improve your overall health without using chemical medications.

Dr. Sebi's theory is that all diseases are caused by too much mucus building up in a specific body area. When you have too much mucus in your lungs, you get pneumonia. If you have too much mucus in your pancreas, it causes diabetes.

He believes that any disease won't exist in an alkaline environment but can happen if your body is too acidic.

Many people claim that his diet improved their health by using his compounds, and the herbal approach to heal the body worked better than any medical approach ever did.

His diet does offer many health benefits. The main one is it can promote weight loss because it restricts processed foods, and you will be eating more plant-based, unprocessed meals. This diet is full of whole fruits and vegetables full of plant compounds, minerals, vitamins, and fiber.

Diets that contain fruits and vegetables are related to oxidative stress and reduced inflammation, along with protecting you against most diseases.

Meatless diets have been linked to lower risks of heart disease and obesity. It also encourages foods that are high in fiber and low in calories. Regularly consuming fruits and vegetables can help protect your body against diseases and reduce inflammation.

If you can switch from your normal diet that is full of fast foods, saturated fats, refined sugars, and grains to Dr. Sebi's diet could help you lose some weight—increasing your intake of grains, vegetables, and fruits while getting rid of pork and beef can decrease your risk of elevated cholesterol, high blood pressure, Type 2 diabetes, heart disease, and cancer. Most people eat way too much sodium, and this diet can drastically reduce this amount. Lowering sodium intake can lower your blood pressure, which reduces your risk of heart disease and stroke.

In one study, people who ate seven servings of fruits and vegetables each day had between 25 and 31 % lower heart disease chance and cancer.

Most Americans don't eat enough produce. During 2017 it was reported that between 9.3 and 12.2 percent met all their recommended daily intake of fruits and vegetables.

Dr. Sebi's diet encourages eating healthy fats like plant oils, seeds, nuts, and whole grain-rich fiber. These foods have a lower risk of developing heart disease.

Any diet that limits processed foods can help you have a better quality of diet.

### Downsides of the Dr. Sebi Diet

While Dr. Sebi's diet helps improve one's health and improve people's quality of life, there can be a few downsides or cons to following the Dr. Sebi diet to the letter.

## Restricted food intake

The Dr. Sebi diet is a modified vegan diet with supplement requirements, in essence. However, while vegan diets already tend to be very restrictive, Dr. Sebi's diet goes even further and has many more restrictions.

Not only are adherents required to avoid animal products altogether and rely wholly on plant-based foods like other vegans, but there are also furthermore specific restrictions. Standard vegan diets, for example, allow any fruit and simply set limits on consumption amounts.

The Dr. Sebi diet, however, goes as far as to bar one from eating certain types of fruit, such as Roma tomatoes or beefsteak tomatoes being restricted, while cherry and plum tomatoes are permitted.

This may lead to certain difficulties when adhering to the diet, as it has been shown that strict diets are more difficult to follow. If one finds it difficult or impossible to follow the diet, they will not benefit from the diet in the first place, defeating the purpose of following the diet.

## Reliance on Supplementation

While supplements are not an inherently bad thing, Dr.Sebi's diet needs to take specific supplements, which can be expensive or hard to source, depending on where one is in the world.

Dr. Sebi's supplements are necessary but not exclusive, meaning that one should also be taking other supplements to make up for any vitamin deficiencies that might have popped up along the way.

That means that one may be confused as to what additional supplements may be necessary. Thus, one who intends to start the Dr.Sebi diet should consult with a nutritionist to design their diet plan according to the Dr.Sebi's rules and determine what additional supplements may be necessary. These supplements necessarily show the inherent flaw in a vegan-based diet, while relying only on plant-based products leads to nutrient deficiencies that need to be made up for supplementation.

For example, protein tends to be hard to come by in vegan diets, and even more so in Dr. Sebi's more restrictive version, protein is an essential macronutrient for us to stay healthy. While nuts are a protein source, it tends to be difficult and impractical to gain all the protein we need just through nut consumption, and thus the need for supplementation. Other things that need to be supplemented are nutrients such as omega 3, iron, calcium, and vitamin B12, which are all necessary to keep the body healthy and balanced but will be difficult to come by when following the Dr. Sebi diet, and thus needing supplementation.

## Risk of Vitamin Deficiencies

One essential thing that we must remember is that while vegetables are extremely nutrient-dense and are, in fact, the best sources for some of the essential nutrients.

Meaning that the body will not worry about getting these nutrients. Some nutrients cannot be provided by an all – plant matter diet, such as Vitamin B – 12, vitamin D, calcium, and certain fatty acids such as the long-chain Omega – 3 fatty acid commonly found in fish, as these nutrients cannot be created by the body using the building blocks it obtains from food, but rather must be obtained directly from an outside source, and one of the better sources and the most easily – absorbable sources, (bioavailable source) would be animal products. As such, vegans are recommended to supplement their diet using appropriate supplementation to ensure that they get all the necessary nutrients to maintain their health and make sure that they keep a balanced diet.

While supplements in the Dr. Sebi diet are crucial and are included in the diet design, the diet itself does not specify food portions and meal design, which means that the supplements may not be enough to make up for nutrient deficiencies.

As the Dr. Sebi diet does not necessarily prescribe what exactly to eat and just prescribes what may be eaten, some people may eat more of one thing and less of another, which may lead to nutrient imbalances, even with the inclusion of the necessary supplements.

One example of this, for example, would be B – 12 nutrient deficiency. Those who are predominantly vegetarian or vegan and do not eat animal products are already at risk of developing a vitamin B – 12 deficiency and thus are recommended to take supplements to cover it. The Dr. Sebi diet supplements may not give enough B – 12 vitamins that one needs, and this is not entirely clear, as the Dr. Sebi diet supplements are necessary but not exclusive, meaning that one should also be taking other supplements to make up for any vitamin deficiencies that might have popped up along the way.

Without consulting a qualified nutritionist, one may run into the risk of developing deficiencies. Thus extra care should be taken when planning and designing a diet plan around Dr. Sebi's diet principles. Another nutrient that those who take the Dr. Sebi diet should watch out for is protein. As with any other vegan diet, protein tends to be in short supply and should be made up of supplementation.

## ASTHMA

*Dr Sebi's herbal tea for asthma*

Dr. Sebi's Ginger Tea

"Ginger tea has been used for asthma for centuries, and we agree that its possible benefits have to do with its anti-inflammatory properties," says Dr. Sebi, who believes that Ginger can help to calm the smooth muscles in the lungs.

Dr. Sebi's Fennel tea

Another herb historically considered to be anti-spasmodic, fennel, can provide some relief to the lungs when taken in tea form.

Green Tea

Green tea, usually containing around 27 mg of caffeine per 8 oz cup, could be worth a try if you're trying to enjoy the mild respiratory benefits of caffeine.

Licorice Tea

Crafted from the root of licorice, this sweet-tasting tea has long been used as a treatment for lung disorders such as asthma.

Licorice causes saliva to thicken and stimulates mucus production, which can gently cover and soothe airways. This effect is incredibly helpful when a nagging cough threatens to cause symptoms of asthma.

*Food to eat*

people who have asthma might be curious as to whether some foods and dietary options may help you control your condition.

At the same time, eating fresh, healthy foods will improve your overall health as well as your symptoms of asthma.

People with asthma can also benefit from eating a well-rounded diet high in fresh fruits and vegetables.

Food comes into play when it applies to allergies, too. Food allergies and food intolerances arise when the immune system overreacts to particular proteins in food. In some instances, this can lead to symptoms of asthma.

## DIABETES

While there is a lot of good advice for diabetics that doctors will share, such as lifestyle changes, there is also a lot of medication that you could end up being prescribed. And let's not get started on how scary it must be to learn how to give yourself insulin injections.

Dr. Sebi's diabetes cure is a super simple plan, and it doesn't cost that much. Very few people wanted to try his plan at first because it required fasting. Most would rather cut off their feet than not eat. Dr. Sebi was able to cure his diabetes with a 27 day fast.

There are a lot of other people who have reported similar results as well. You can find a lot of videos on YouTube, where people talk about having cured their diabetes with Dr. Sebi's plan.

Like with the STD treatments, the goal is to rid the body of excess mucus. For diabetics, the excess mucus is found in the pancreatic duct. Dr. Sebi's own mother started fasting to help her diabetes, and after 57 days, she was cured.

During your fast, you should drink water, and you can also have herbal tea. A great herbal tea to drink is a combination of burdock, black walnut leaf, red raspberry, and elderberry. Use a tablespoon of each and mix them into one and a half liters of spring water. Boil and steep for 15 minutes. Take this off the heat and mix in another half liter of water. Strain out the herbs and place to the side to use the next day. Store the tea in the fridge and drink as much as you want during the day.

A lot of people, when they hear the word fast, assume that means they can't take anything by mouth. But that's not Dr. Sebi's fast. See, when Dr. Sebi fasted to cure his diabetes, he would take three green plus tablets each day and drink sea moss tea, spring water, and tamarind juice. You don't have to drink tamarind juice, though. Any juice that is on the approved list of foods is okay. It must be fresh juice, though. You don't want pre-made juice with a bunch of added sugars.

Once you have fasted for a while, and your body will let you know when you have had enough, you will then need to start the Dr. Sebi approved diet plan. Along with that, you should also think about taking black seeds, mulberry leaves, and fig leaves. Research on black seeds has found that taking as little as two teaspoons of the powder each day can reverse diabetes.

Figleaves are the top alternative medicine for diabetes on the market today. Mulberry leaves are a common treatment for diabetes in the Middle East. These can be made into a tea, and you can mix in some black seeds as well.

Some other foods that you should consider adding to your diet are ginseng, okra, ginger, fenugreek, red clover, swiss chard, avocado, and bitter melon.

# HIV

HIV has been, and for many, still is one of the scariest STDs you can contract. HIV stands for human immunodeficiency virus and can lead to AIDS, acquired immunodeficiency syndrome. There are a lot of "beliefs" about HIV/AIDS, most of which are unfounded and are caused by ill-informed gossip.

HIV harms the immune system by killing the white blood cells that you need to fight off infections. This places a person at risk for developing some serious infections and certain types of cancers. Once HIV reaches its final stages, it becomes AIDS, but not everybody who contracts HIV will develop AIDS. For a long time, people thought HIV and AIDS were one and the same, but they aren't.

The most common way for HIV to be spread is through unprotected sex with an HIV positive person. It can also be spread through shared drug needles or contact with the blood of an infected person. Women are also able to give it to their children during childbirth or pregnancy.

Some of the first signs of an HIV infection could be flu-like symptoms and swollen glands. These could also come and go within a couple of weeks to a month. You may not experience severe symptoms until several months or years later. You could experience a primary infection or acute HIV. Most of those who have been infected will develop flu-like symptoms within a couple of months after exposure. This is what is known as the primary infection. Some of the most common signs of the primary infection are:

- Swollen lymph glands, mostly in the neck
- Painful mouth sores and sore throat
- Rash
- Joint pain and muscle aches
- Headache
- Fever

It is possible these symptoms could be so mild that they may go unnoticed. However, how much of the virus you have in your bloodstream is very high during this stage. This is why the infection will spread more easily during this time than once you reach the next stage.

The next stage is clinical latent infection or chronic HIV. For some, they will still have swollen lymph nodes. Otherwise, there aren't any really specific symptoms and signs. HIV will say in the body and your white blood cells. If one does not get diagnosed and receive some sort of therapy, this stage can last for ten years. Some people will develop severe secondary diseases a lot sooner.

Then there is the symptomatic HIV infection. As the virus starts to grow and kill off your immune cells, you could start to develop chronic signs or mild infections, like:

- Shingles
- Oral yeast infections
- Weight loss
- Diarrhea
- Swollen lymph nodes
- Fatigue
- Fever

With better antiviral medicines, most HIV patients don't develop AIDS. If left untreated, HIV will normally turn into AIDS within 10 years. Once AIDS develops, the immune system has already been severely damaged. It places a person at a higher risk of opportunistic cancers or infections, which are a disease that a person with a healthy immune system wouldn't have to worry about. The most common signs and symptoms of these secondary infections could include:

- Skin bumps or rashes
- Weight loss
- Persistent and unexplained fatigue
- Persistent white spots or odd lesions in your mouth or on the tongue
- Chronic diarrhea
- Recurring fever
- Soaking night sweats

HIV can only be spread through sex or contact with blood, or from mother to child during childbirth, pregnancy, or breastfeeding. When it comes to contact with blood, the blood has to entire a mucous membrane, such as the nose, mouth, anus, or vagina. Simply touching infected blood won't spread HIV, and once the blood is dried, it isn't dangerous.

The common ways for HIV to be spread is:

- Sex – This is one of the most common ways for it to be spread. You can get infected by having unprotected oral, anal, or vaginal sex with an infected person whose vaginal secretions, semen, or blood enters your body. The virus is able to enter into the body through mouth sores, or through small tears that can occur in the vagina or rectum during sex.
- Blood Transfusions – At one time, people could end up contracting HIV through a blood transfusion. Nowadays, American blood banks and hospitals screen the blood for HIV antibodies, so the odds of this happening now are small.
- Sharing Needles – The second most common way for HIV to be spread is by sharing contaminated intravenous drug paraphernalia.
- Breastfeeding, Pregnancy, or Delivery – Mothers who are HIV-positive can pass it onto their babies. Mothers who make sure that they are receiving treatment are able to lower the risk of passing it along.

Modern medicine has yet to find a cure for HIV, but there are a lot of medications that can help to fight the HIV infection and lower a person's risk of infecting other people. People who are able to get treated early are able to live a long life with the disease, which has not always been the case.

Treatments for HIV are called antiretroviral therapy or ART. The various classes of drugs work by blocking the virus in various ways. ART is a recommended treatment for everybody, no matter what their T cell levels are.

Most HIV treatments will require you to take several different pills at certain times during the day for the remainder of your life. Every medication will come with its own side effects that you will have to get used to. It is very important that you go to regular check-ups with your doctor to keep an eye on your health and your treatment progress. Some of the common side effects of treatment include:

- High blood sugar levels
- Abnormal cholesterol levels
- Breakdown of muscle tissue
- Bone loss or weakened bones
- Heart disease
- Diarrhea, nausea, or vomiting

As you age, there are some age-related health issues that can become more difficult to manage. There are medications that you might have been given otherwise, for age-related diseases, that don't interact very well with your HIV medications. This will involve speaking with your doctor and monitoring every situation.

Besides medical treatments, a person will also be advised to make certain lifestyle changes to help.

- Take off Your Pets – There are some animals that carry parasites that can end up causing infections in those who have HIV. Cat feces can end up causing toxoplasmosis. Salmonella is found in reptiles. Birds can also pass along histoplasmosis or cryptococcus. It is vital you wash your hands extremely well after you have handled your pets or cleaned their litter box.
- Make Sure You Get Immunizations – It is often suggested that HIV-positive individuals receive regular flu and pneumonia vaccinations to prevent secondary diseases. It is also important that the vaccines are not live viruses because these can be very dangerous for those with weakened immune systems.
- Stay Away from Raw Eggs, Meat, and More – Foodborne illnesses are more dangerous for people who have HIV. HIV-positive individuals should never eat anything that is raw or unpasteurized.
- Eat Healthy Foods – Fresh veggies and fruits, as well as whole grains, can help to keep and HIV-positive individuals strong and healthy and can help support the immune system.

The treatment goes beyond the actual treatment of the disease. It also involved coping and support. Getting a diagnosis like HIV is devastating. The financial, emotional, and social consequences of HIV can make it a lot harder to cope with the illness, and this is true for those closest to you as well.

Dr. Sebi offers an alternative to modern medicine when it comes to treating HIV. He believes that cleaning the mucus buildup in the lymphatic system and blood can help HIV.

Dr. Sebi didn't create something specifically to treat HIV/AIDS or any specific disease. Instead, he came up with compounds meant to cleanse the body and provide essential nutrition.

We are constantly trying to find any means to remain hydrated to deal with our suffocation through animal products, medical-chemicals, starch, and sugar.

More than 40 herbs have been developed by Dr. Sebi to nourish and cleanse your body of inflammation. You don't need to travel so far, even though many people will go to Usha Village in Honduras to receive HIV/AIDS treatment. All you have to do is eat only alkaline foods and follow the dietary guidelines.

The immune system is made up of the skin, blood, and lymphatic system. You must follow a rigorous diet in order to get rid of the mucus in these places. It will take much longer to mend if you don't. You should only eat green, leafy plants to aid in healing,

The list of permitted foods also includes peppers, spices, and mushrooms, all of which you may consume. When beginning to follow this diet, it's crucial to remember to drink a gallon of water day and engage in some modest activity. It's a good idea to prepare a gallon jug for the day at the beginning of the day, and you can add any water consumed for teas. Red clover tea should be substituted for chamomile.

You should start by treating your iron deficiency because your immune system needs a lot of it. For ten days, you must consume one bottle of either Bio Ferro or Iron Plus every day. Once you start your therapeutic program, you simply need to take two to three spoonfuls. You can also have a cup of bromide tea every day at noon and at night.

After that, you should begin taking a variety of various supplements for the first ten days. Some will choose to take them all, while others will just pick a handful.

You can improve HIV/AIDS if you start eating like Dr. Sebi and start taking his supplements. Nevertheless, it is still advisable to visit your doctor regularly for monitoring. You are free to take the prescription drugs that your doctor has given you while doing this. It's vital to take your supplements one hour before you take your prescriptions, as you'll see in the nutritional guide. This enables the supplements to benefit your body and repair it from any negative side effects that the medications may have.

Last but not least, you may have observed that Dr. Sebi's HIV and herpes treatments are rather similar. Although there are some variations, most therapies will proceed in a similar manner. So, by starting the therapy for one illness, you will be assisting in the prevention of other illnesses.

## HAIR LOSS

Alopecia or hair loss is a problem for children, women, and men. Treatments include hair restoration techniques, hair replacements, or medicines like Rogaine and Propecia.

There is hair everywhere on the human body except the soles of the feet and the palms of the hand. We do have some hairs that are so fine that they are hard to see. Hair is made from a protein known as keratin. This is made in the hair follicles on the outer layer of our skin. When the follicles make new hair, the old get pushed out of the skin's surface of a rate of six inches each year. The hair that is visible to the naked eye is actually a string of dead keratin cells. A normal adult head will have around 100,000 to 150,000 hairs. It will lose around 100 of these every single day. When you find some stray hair in your hairbrush isn't anything to be worried about.

## Signs of Hair Loss

These signs will vary between children, women, and men. But people of any sex or age might notice some more hair being collected in your shower drain or hairbrush.

Some signs of hair loss in men might include:

- A semi-circle shaped pattern that exposes the crown
- Receding hairline
- Thinner hair

Signs of hair loss in women:

- Thinning of the hair especially at the crown

Signs of hair loss in young adults and children:

- Excessive shedding of hair after stress, anemia, rapid weight loss, drug treatments, and illnesses
- Incomplete hair loss or patches of broken hairs on the eyebrows or scalp
- Total loss of hair over all the body
- Sudden loss of hair in patches

When to call your doctor:

- Our child or yourself have suffered an unexplained hair loss on any body part
- Your child is pulling or rubbing out their hair
- Your child has incomplete hair loss or broken hairs on their eyebrows or scalp
- Your child or yourself has a sudden loss of hair in patches

## Treatments

There are some remedies that promise to restore hair to a balding head, and some of these have been used since ancient times. Most women and men who have thinning hair can't do much to reverse this process. Most people will turn to weaving, hairpieces, and wigs after they lost their hair from drug treatments or surgery. Some might get a tattoo to simulate eyelashes or eyebrows. There are some drugs that can slow down hair loss, and there are some alternative treatments that can help the remaining hairs' health, but there isn't one treatment that will replace a complete head of hair.

Some people could benefit from these treatments:

- Janus Kinase Inhibitors

This is a class of immunomodulators is showing some promises in the clinical studies that treat alopecia areata

- Lasers

Home-based and office laser devices have been successful in stimulating hair growth.

- Diphencyprone

This is a sensitizing agent that is used topically and only occasionally to stimulate the hair growth for people who have alopecia areata.

- Anthralin or Drithocreme

This is a medication that is used topically to control the inflammation around the base of the hair follicles. It has been used to treat conditions like alopecia areata.

- Corticosteroids

In some cases of alopecia areata, a person's hair loss will resolve itself spontaneously. In most cases of alopecia areata which is an autoimmune disorder, is what causes a person's hair to fall out in clumps. Some doctors will try to speed up recovery by prescribing topical corticosteroids or shots directly in the areas of hair loss. This treatment might be a bit painful and might cause some skin to thin at the injection sites. Prednisone could be effective for alopecia areata, but the side effects could include menstrual problems, acne, metabolic abnormalities, and weight gain. Any positive effects are normally just temporary.

## Prevention

Even though there isn't a total cure for balding, you could protect your hair from being damaged and leading to the thinning of the hair.

Most people put a lot of stress on how their hair looks. Chemical cosmetics, hair straightening products, tight braids, permanents, hair dyes, hot curlers, and hair dryers could cause thinning, brittle, and dry hair.

In order to prevent damage to your hair, do the following:

- Brush Right

Brushing your hair properly could do the same damage to your hair as any other product. Using the right brush, apply gentle pressure to the scalp and bring the brush down to the tips of the hair to distribute the natural oils into the hair. You have to work gently and don't brush your hair when it is wet. This is the time when your hair is most fragile. When your hair is wet, you need to use a wide-tooth comb.

- Pick the Right Products

Use a shampoo that is right for your type of hair. If you like curling your hair, pick sponge rollers as they won't damage your hair. Use a natural-bristle brush that is slightly stiff. It won't break or tear the hair.

- Be Natural

Try to leave your hair its natural texture and color. If this isn't an option, give your hair time to recover between chemical treatments or blowouts. Don't tightly braid your hair.

## Hair Loss for Women

The easiest way to think about how your hair grows is to compare it to a garden. How well your garden grows, all depends on what happens underground.

Just like a garden, a normal growing cycle should produce a product, which is your hair. Hair growth cycles are important since if they don't work properly, this is a reason we lose our hair.

Chemicals, infection, illness, and medications can interfere with this cycle, and they can stop hair from growing properly.

Even though hair loss might seem more prominent in men, women are just as likely to have thinning or no hair. Most women will see it when they reach their 50s and 60s, but it could happen at any age for many reasons.

- Ways to Grow

As stated above, the hair will grow in three stages: telogen, catagen, and anagen. Around 90 percent of all the hair on your head is in the anagen stage.. The catagen stage usually lasts about two to three weeks. During this time, the hair follicle will shrink. In the telogen stage, the hair will rest. This will last about two to four months.

Most of the time, the hair will be growing. About ten percent of the strands will be in the resting or transition stage at the same time. Hair will grow around six inches each year.

- Losing Hair

Many people will lose about 50 to 100 strands every day. When you wash your hair, you could lose about 250 strands. Don't ever stop washing your hair to try to keep it. It is going to fall out eventually.

For people who don't count their hair each day, there are ways to see if your hair is being lost faster or thinning. Women will notice the difference faster than men. When you wake up each morning, look at your pillow, there might be a large amount of hair on your pillow. Each time you comb your hair, you might notice a large amount being left in the comb or brush.

There are other cues that you could look for. Even though men's hair normally recedes from the crown or forehead, women will notice the thinning on the top half or third of their scalp. Their frontal line normally stays intact. Women might see their part getting wider, or they might see more scalp when they pull their hair back.

There are ways your doctor can make a diagnosis. Blood work will be taken to rule out autoimmune diseases or thyroid problems aren't to blame.

- Genes

There are other ways to diagnose your problem, and that is by listening and looking. Just take some time to look at your ancestors. If some of them have similar or even greater amounts of hair loss, you can expect to look like them one day. Your doctor can use a magnifying glass to look at the scalp to see if your follicles are in different sizes. These are some good signs of female pattern baldness. This is also known as androgenetic alopecia.

This condition is hereditary and affects around 30 million women. It is the most common type of hair loss. It happens in about 50 percent of all women. It normally shows up in their late 50s or 60s, but it could happen any time even as early as their teenage years.

Every time a normal hair follicle is lost, it gets replaced by one that is the same size. Women who have female pattern baldness, the new hair will be thinner and finer. Basically, it becomes a miniaturized version of itself. Your follicles are getting smaller, and they will eventually stop growing.

- Medical Conditions

If all your hair follicles are the same size, or if you have a sudden loss in hair, it is probably caused by something more than just heredity, such as a medical problem.

There are many conditions that could cause hair loss. The most common are anemia, thyroid problems, and pregnancy. Others might include seborrheic dermatitis, psoriasis, PCOS or polycystic ovary syndrome, and autoimmune diseases.

Even though there is a link between hair loss and menopause, there isn't a direct correlation. It might be that hair loss and menopause just happen around the same age. Other reasons might include too much vitamin A, drastic weight loss in a short amount of time, intense illness, surgery, or extreme stress. Hair loss could happen in just a couple of weeks, or it might take six months.

- Take It Easy

Another way that thinning hair is self-inflicted is people who wear their hair in extremely tight braids or cornrows. Everything that a woman does to manipulate their hair, flat irons, blow dryers, bad brushes, chemical treatments could cause breakage and damage. These include too much brushing and aggressively towel drying when your hair is wet.

For most of these problems, the hair will grow back, or the loss could be changed with medical treatments. You need to see a dermatologist if you think something is wrong. The sooner you start treatment, the more chances you will have for improving your hair growth.

## Caring for Thinning Hair

You can lose hair for many different reasons. Medicines and illnesses could cause hair loss. Hair loss could be inherited. Usually,the hair will thin due to being fine-textured, or you have used too many harsh chemicals on your hair, and it begins to break easily.

These tips can protect your hair, add volume, and prevent more hair loss:

- Pick a Style that Works for You

Blow dryers aren't a problem if you keep the heat low. Be extremely careful about placing heat onto your hair. Curling irons and flat irons could damage your hair and cause breakage.

- Shampoo Hair When Needed

In order to protect your hair, it is best to only shampoo your hair when it gets dirty. Since fine hair will get dirty faster, people who have fine hair will need to shampoo more often, although fine hair will break easier. Fine-textured hair will benefit from getting a good shampoo and some conditioner that will build volume.

- Use Volumizers

Most hair products that build volume will contain paraffin or beeswax. This isn't good for hair since it can build up and make your hair break. If you buy your products at a salon, they will actually help. They don't damage the hair or weigh it down. You can apply mousse at the roots for some support. You can start blow drying at the roots. Apply some pressure gently with a brush to create some volume. You can use a finishing spray to hold it in place.

## *How Dr. Sebi Reversed Alopecia*

Dr. Sebi has constantly shared all his discoveries about food. He created a program that was found to be "consistent with the African genetic structure." The food he recommends is not hybrids. Hybrid foods need starch to get bound together. Starch is basically an acid.

Dr. Sebi's diet is based on the knowledge that foods could influence our body's pH levels. This means all the foods we eat could make our bodies more basic or more acidic. Because diseases thrive in acidic environments where mucus starts to spread in the body, this will keep oxygen away from our vital organs. He thought that you could reverse this process by getting rid of starch and blood from the diet.

Should you try Dr. Sebi's diet? Well, only you can answer that question. He was a true believer that there wasn't any book that could give you the knowledge that your own experiments and discovery could. Even though he was and is still trusted by many, it is important for you to do your own research before changing your diet. If a diet requires any drastic changes to how you look at food, you need to ask yourself some important questions.

I have asked myself: "If my grandmother has lived for 100 years and is still going strong, and I watch her eat pickled pig's feet, what does this mean for me?"

You have to challenge yourself with some questions that you don't know the answers to. If you think that Dr. Sebi's diet is something that might help you and you want to try it, begin with some baby steps. Do a lot of research online and find support groups. Find some recipes that were inspired by Dr. Sebi and give them a try. If you have to change them up until you get the diet down, that is fine. The main thing is to do your research and listen to your body. This will make your experience better, and it will make you feel more confident in changing your lifestyle.

# HYPERTENSION

High blood pressure is initiated when the blood flowing to the arteries is high due to the consumption of foods capable of clogging the arteries' wall. An act that results in pressure through the arteries during the distribution of blood flow. Peradventure, the arteries' walls become narrow and hardened due to excessive plague caused by poor eating habits, blood flow in the passageway of the arteries suppresses. Worthy of note is that as an individual gets older, the arteries get hardened bit by bit, and a bad diet will triple the possibility of high blood pressure.

Some of the numerous causes of high blood pressure are:

- Bad diet
- Tobacco intake
- Stress
- Excess coffee intake
- Fried and processed foods
- Over-eating
- Aging

## Natural Remedies for Hypertension

Every medication for high blood pressure on the market mimics water. To be effective, you must consume twice your weight in pounds of water every day. Just why so much water? You may inquire. Water, on the other hand, thins the blood and eases the flow through the arteries.

A daily intake of five different types of fruits, including vegetables, will stop the arteries from being blocked with too much plaque. Vegetables and fruits that contain a high percentage of antioxidants protect the artery walls from plaque deposits. Such fruits include peaches, oranges, cabbage, seeded grapes, and tomatoes.

Foods high in potassium help lower recurrent hypertension because it helps the body eliminate excess salt. Fruits that include fiber are also very beneficial for people who have high blood pressure since they lower the blood pressure while also eliminating waste from the artery walls.

High blood pressure after eating:

Food-related high blood pressure knowledge is important as knowing what foods to eat and avoiding is detrimental to the blood pressure level. No one wants to get high blood pressure from eating like everybody else.

Here are some things to avoid:

- Avoid overeating even the healthiest of food.
- Avoid salty foods as much as possible as they transform into plaque in the artery walls. In essence, avoid baking soda, sodas, soy sauce, and meat tenderizers.
- Never eat canned foods.
- Eliminate dairy products such as sodium, cheese, and alcohol after your diet.
- Avoid every other type of rice except wild and brown

The herbs listed below are recommended by Dr. Sebi as they support opening the blood vessels, exposed the arteries' walls, and eliminate plaques from the wall of arteries. These herbs are alkaline, high in iron and other minerals. They are not hearsays; they have been medically proved to be effective as blood pressure medication.

Some of these herbs include:

- Fennel
- Oregano
- Basil
- Yellow dock
- Cayenne

## About Hypertension

If the arteries' walls were to be clogged or packed with plagues, blood flow would become restricted as it pumps from the heart to the aorta. When the arteries create pressure in a situation like this, the blood pressure becomes higher than it should be, resulting in hypertension (high blood pressure).

Poor diet is the leading cause of high blood pressure in the United States as it has been reported that over 85 percent of reported high blood pressure cases are rooted in a poor diet. More than any other race in the United States, African Americans reported more high blood pressure cases. High blood pressure is a channel to other diseases such as kidney diseases, strokes, scarlet fever, large heart, typhoid fever, artery coronary diseases, and tonsillitis. These diseases are rampant among African Americans who have a hypertensive health history.

To be certain of your blood pressure, you will need a blood pressure gauge for accuracy. This gauge is often called a sphygmomanometer. It records two basic types of information: the first being systolic, which the higher reading is, while the second is diastolic, which the lower reading is.

Consequently, the diastolic high blood pressure is less problematic than the systolic high blood pressure readings. The systolic shows the blood pressure built as it is being pumped through the passageways in the aorta's arteries. The blood pressure is high when your systolic reading is high due to the artery walls being clogged, thereby limiting blood flows. A regular systolic hypertension reading is usually among 120 – 150 millimeters. On the other hand, a high understanding is 140/190; the sign of a systolic hypertension reading is over 180/115.

Symptoms of High Blood Pressure:

According to Dr. Sebi, high blood pressure symptoms can be likened to "navy seal snipers", as there are no signs that a person's blood pressure is high.

The few noticeable pointers of high blood pressure have always been:

- Difficulty breathing
- Blurry vision
- Rapid pulses
- Constant headache

My mother, when alive, had high blood pressure. She once told me that her blood pressure symptoms are dizziness and that her pulse gets fast often.

# LUPUS

Having lupus isn't a joking matter. What makes this disease even worse is the way health care professionals work with lupus patients. Some doctors want to kill your immune system with chemotherapy or begin giving you shots of concentrated starch, which is a lot worse than alcohol. They might as well just put lupus in the same boat as AIDS. The main reason that it hasn't been considered as AIDS is that it doesn't shatter the immune system. The truth of the matter is that for people who have lupus, their immune system is so screwed up that you would be better off not having one. This is why I said it might as well be AIDS.

- What About Lupus?

What has Dr. Sebi taught us about lupus? Your central nervous system has been compromised because there is a yeast infection that no one has addressed right. The cells' mucous membranes are constantly being attacked and turned into pus, and mucus contributes to the cells being deprived of oxygen. Because the cells are exposed and our bodies are stressed with the effort of just trying to function properly, our central nervous system needs some serious help.

- Living Without a Central Nervous System

The life of our cells and nerves that are responsible for sending signals through our bodies have been challenged and diminished as more cells get compromised, and this contributes to more mucus forming in other parts of our bodies. Our bodies are still smart enough to know that it needs to be cleansed since mucus is stopping the cells from doing their job correctly. This will soon keep your organs from doing what they are supposed to do. This causes your pain receptors to go on overload to tell you that something is wrong with the body. Your brain and body want you to quit eating specific foods, and you should know what you need to quit eating. When it seems like your organs don't want to work right, they then start acting like an enemy rather than a friend. Can you guess what your immune system is saying about all this? What do you think your immune system is going to do? It is going to start attacking everything in sight. Now your organs are being attacked. They can't fix themselves anymore, and you can't even get a good night's sleep.

- Why Worry About the Nervous System?

Our bodies need to be able to protect and repair the central nervous system because it helps protect our immune system. They do things at the same time as long as our bodies are producing dopamine naturally. Our bodies can instinctively and immediately protect themselves by sending out phagocyte cells to protect and defend it. It already has these cells place throughout our bodies. Phagocyte cells called neutrophils are what begin attacking your organs. This causes them to die and turn into pus or mucus. We have more of these cells in our bodies than any other kind of phagocytes. These stationary cells called macrophages will begin eating right where they are at. They are only following orders, and they don't know what is good and what is bad. Pain receptors begin going off. But they aren't finished yet. Our central nervous system has some tough guys in the blood. They are called our "natural killer cells." Just imagine what is going to happen when these get confused about who their enemy is? These cells patrol the lymphatic and blood systems, just trying to find any abnormal cells. They will kill off healthy cells faster than they can erode away.

- You Now Have a Compromised Central Nervous System

Your body is confused, and your immune system sets off a fever so that your metabolism gets faster trying to repair everything quickly. This fever begins attracting histamines to areas that have been damaged so they can help call the phagocytes. Now, your body feels as if it has the flu. By this time, the immune system is using the fever to help heal; it is also calling the bones to help trigger leukocytosis. This is when the bone marrow begins producing more neutrophils to help fight. Now, while all this is happening, guess who was supposed to be making sure that everything is being done correctly and that the right enemies have been found: your lymphatic system.

Your lymphatic and immune systems are one and the same. It is supposed to clean up the dirty cells and make them all clean and new. If it fails to do this, your blood pressure is going to drop, your lungs will fill with fluid, your ankles are going to start swelling, and your body just wants to give up and die.

- How to Handle Lupus?

You get rid of it the same way you get rid of AIDS, cancer, and tumors. You use the Bio-mineral balance along with Intra-cellular chelation. These require you to eat an extremely strict diet. Intra-cellular chelation just means that you are going to clean your cells; every single cell that makes up your central nervous system and organs. You won't just be cleaning your organs but every single cell that makes the organ. Why do you need to do this? If you have cancer present in your body, it is telling you that you have a high level of acid in the body. This is a very high level of mitosis. Mitosis is a cell that eats the tissues and organs. This happens when there is a presence of acid. We have to nourish every part of our bodies at the same time. Disease requires us to nourish our bodies back to health. We need to give them Bio-mineral Balance. This along with the Intra-cellular chelation, will bring our bodies back to the way they were before.

So, what exactly are we going to do:

- We give our bodies electric cell nutrition
- We get rid of the mucus
- We stay away from foods that create mucus, hybrid foods, synthetic sugars, and starches
- We fast

## Support and Coping

If you have been diagnosed with lupus, you are probably going to have a lot of painful feelings about your disease from extreme frustration to fear. There are challenges to living with lupus that can increase the risk of mental health problems like low self-esteem, stress, anxiety, or depression. To help you cope, you can try:

- Connecting With Others

You can try talking to others who have lupus. You can find people through message boards, community centers, and support groups. Other people who have lupus could give you unique support since they are facing the same frustrations and obstacles that you are facing.

- Time for Yourself

You can cope with the stress by taking time for yourself. Use this time to write in a journal, listen to music, meditate, or read. Find an activity that will renew and calm you.

- Get Support

Find support from your family and friends. Talk about your lupus with family and friends and explain how they could help you when you have flares. Lupus is a frustrating disease for loved one since they can't feel or see it, and you might not look like you are sick.

- Educate Yourself

You can ask your nurse or doctor for reputable sources for more information. The more you know about your disease, the more confident you are going to feel about your treatments.

## Your Appointment

When you see your health care provider, they might refer you to a specialist to get a diagnosis and for your treatments for any immune disorders and inflammatory joint problems.

Since lupus symptoms mimic other health conditions, you might need to have some patience while you are waiting on your diagnosis. Your doctor has to rule out other illnesses before they diagnosis lupus. You might need to see many specialists like a neurologist, hematologist, or nephrologist. It all depends on what symptoms you are experiencing.

## Things You Can Do

Before you go to your appointment, write down answers to these questions:

- What supplements and medications do you regularly take?
- Have your siblings or parents been diagnosed with an autoimmune disease or lupus?
- When did the symptoms start? Do they go away and come back?

You might want to write down some questions for your doctor like:

- Do I need to see a specialist?
- Are there any restrictions I need to adhere to while waiting for a diagnosis?
- What type of test are you recommending?
- If these don't point to a specific cause, what other tests am I going to need?
- What are some of the causes of my condition or symptoms?
- I am thinking about getting pregnant. What do I need to do? Are there certain medicines that I can't use if I am pregnant?

Never hesitate to ask any question that might pop into your mind while you are at your doctor's office or if there is something they bring you that you don't understand.

## What to Expect from the Doctor

Your doctor is going to ask you a lot of questions. You need to be ready to answer them. This will leave you plenty of time to go over the things you want to spend time on. Your doctor could ask:

- Do you plan on getting pregnant, or are you pregnant?
- Do you have any other medical problems?
- Do your symptoms limit your ability to function at home, work, or school? How much do they limit you?
- Are you having problems concentrating or with your memory?
- When you are in the cold, do your fingers get uncomfortable, numb, or pale?
- Do you get rashes when you are out in the sun?

## Outlook

People who were diagnosed in the past normally wouldn't survive more than five years. Now, treatment could increase their lifespan. Effective therapy helps you manage lupus, so you can live a healthy, active life. As researchers learn more about genetics, doctors hope they will soon be able to find lupus in earlier stages. This makes it easy to prevent complications before they actually happen. Some people decide to join clinical trials because this can give them access to different medications.

# PCOS TREATMENT

Polycystic ovary syndrome (PCOS) is a hormonal disorder that affects women within their reproductive age range. That is from 15 to 44 years. Research shows that 2.2 and 26.7 percent of women within the range of 15-44 years of age have PCOS, and about 70% of the women don't even know they are suffering from PCOS.

## What Are The Causes Of PCOS?

Today, most doctors believe that PCOS is caused by the excess of male hormone (androgen). Things like insulin resistance, genetics, and inflammation causes women to produce more androgen hormone, so they are usually linked to PCOS.

## Insulin resistance

If we look at the numbers of women suffering from PCOS, approximately 70% of them have issues with their cells trying to use insulin properly. So, if their cells cannot use insulin, the body will demand more insulin. As the pancreas keeps producing more insulin, the ovaries will be forced to produce more male hormones, leading to obesity or type 2 diabetes.

## Genes

Research shows that PCOS can be transferred from one mother to the other.

## Inflammation

When you don't watch your weight, you might suffer from inflammation, and research shows that excess inflammation can lead to excess production of androgen hormone by women. However, Dr. Sebi state that there is only one disease, which is the compromising of the mucous membrane, and wherever the mucous is compromised, determine the sickness that will manifest and when it is in the ovaries, it is called PCOS.

What Are The Symptoms Of PCOS?

Some women might be lucky to experience some symptoms around the time of their first period, whereas others may only get to know after gaining a lot of weight and others when they find it difficult to get pregnant.

However, the symptoms that one will experience when suffering from PCOS include:

- Irregular or unusual periods: if you have PCOS, one of the symptoms is that you might only experience eight periods in a year because of the delay in-between period.
- Heavy bleeding: because of the uterine lining that will build up for a longer period without experiencing a period, when it comes, it will be heavier than a normal period.
- Hair growth: The women will show some masculine features like hair growth on their body and face because of the excess male hormone. Research has that more than 70% of women suffering from PCOS experience or have hair on their face and body.
- Break out like acne: The male hormones allow men skin to be oilier than usual, which will lead to breakouts on the face, chest etc.
- Weight gain or obesity: research shows that more than 80% of women with PCOS are having excess body weight (obese).

- Hair loss: some women with PCOS experience that their scalp's hair will become thinner and fall out.
- Sometimes Headaches: hormonal change can lead to headaches in some women.

## How Do I Know If I Have PCOS?

If you experience any two out of these three symptoms, you should go and see your doctor or lab technician for an ultrasound scan.

The three symptoms are:

1. High level of androgen hormone.
2. Experiencing heavy menstrual flow or irregular menstrual cycles.
3. If there are cysts in your ovaries

Meeting with your doctor or lab technician, you will be asked some questions like:

- Do you have symptoms like acne on your face?
- Are you experiencing an overweight gain?
- Are you experiencing hair growth on your face and body?
- Have you missed your periods, and you're not pregnant?
- Have you been trying to get pregnant for more than 12 months without any good news?
- Do you have diabetes symptoms like excessive thirst or hunger, possibly blurred vision, or unexplained weight loss?

Once you are experiencing any other symptoms, the lab technicians will recommend an ultrasound scan for confirmation.

## What Are The Complications Of Suffering From PCOS?

There are some severe complications that one can suffer from if she is suffering from PCOS.

For example:

1. If you are having a higher-than-normal level of androgen hormone as a woman, there is a tendency that your fertility will be affected. To be pregnant, you have to ovulate. Women suffering from PCOS do not ovulate regularly, and women who do not ovulate regularly often have issues with releasing enough eggs for fertilization.
2. Metabolic syndrome: research has it that more than 80% of women that are suffering from PCOS are suffering from an obese or overweight issue, which is one of the major cause of; high blood sugar level, high blood pressure, and low HDL and high LDL that increase the risk of heart disease, diabetes, and stroke.
3. Women who are overweight or suffering from obesity always suffer repeated pauses in breathing during the night, interrupting their sleep. Women with PCOS have the chance to suffer sleep apnea 5-10 times higher than normal women suffering from obesity without PCOS.
4. Women who do not ovulate (shedding uterine lining) regularly because they are suffering from PCOS will build up the lining, which will increase the chances of endometrial cancer.
5. Unwanted hair growths from women, and hormonal changes have the potential to affect women's emotions negatively.

*What Can I Do To Treat And Prevent PCOS?*

According to the late Dr. Sebi, there have never been two diseases in this world. The only one disease is the compromising of the mucous membrane, which is caused by our dieting plan and the only way to get rid of PCOS is by eliminating mucus from the entire body and eating the alkaline diet, which will help the body to reverse it to its original alkaline state where sickness cannot withstand.

## STD TREATMENTS

STDs, which stands for sexually transmitted diseases, are still fairly prevalent even though there are well-known ways to prevent them. There are several diseases that fall into the category of STDs and are spread by sexual intercourse, but can be spread through other manners. The most common STDs are trichomoniasis, syphilis, some types of hepatitis, gonorrhea, genital warts, genital herpes, Chlamydia, and HIV.

At one time, STDs were referred to as venereal diseases. They are some of the most common contagious infections. About 65 million Americans have been diagnosed with an incurable STD. Every year, 20 million new cases occur, and about half of these are in people aged 15 to 24. All of these can have long-term implications.

These are serious illnesses that need to be treated. Some of them are considered incurable and can be deadly, such as HIV. Learning more about these diseases can provide you with knowledge on how to protect yourself.

STDs can be spread through oral, vaginal, and anal sex. Trichomoniasis is able to be contracted through contact with a moist or damp object, like toilet seats, wet clothing, or towels, although it is mostly spread through sexual contact. People who are at a higher risk of STDs include:

- Those who have more than one sexual partner.
- Those who trade sex for drugs or money.
- Those who share needles for drug use.
- Those who don't use condoms during sex.
- Those who have sex with a person who has had several partners.

Herpes and HIV are the two STDs that are chronic conditions that modern medicine can cure, but can only manage. Hepatitis B can sometimes become chronic. Unfortunately, you sometimes don't find out that you have an STD until it has damaged your reproductive organs, heart, vision, or other organs. STDs can also weaken the immune system, which leaves you vulnerable to contracting other diseases. Chlamydia and gonorrhea can cause pelvic inflammatory disease, and this can leave women unable to conceive. It is also able to kill you. If an STD is passed onto a newborn, the baby could face permanent damage, or it could kill them.

*Causes of STDs*

In terms of modern medicine, STDs are caused by all types of infection. Syphilis, gonorrhea, and Chlamydia are bacteria. Hepatitis B, genital warts, genital herpes, and HIV are all viral. Parasites cause trichomoniasis.

The STD germs live within vaginal secretions, blood semen, and, in some cases, saliva. The majority of the organisms will be spread through oral, anal, or vaginal sex, but some, like with genital warts and genital herpes, can be spread simply through skin-to-skin contact. Hepatitis B is able to be spread through sharing personal items, like razors or toothbrushes.

*Prevention*

The most obvious step in healing for STDs is to not get one in the first place. The first tip people give in preventing STDs is to not have sex, or at least avoid sex with people who have genital discharge, rash, sores, or other symptoms. The only time you should have unprotected sex is if you and your partner are only having sex with one another, and you have both tests negative for STDs in the last six months. Otherwise, you need to make sure you:

- Use condoms whenever you have sex. If you need a lubricant, make sure that it is one that is water-based. Condoms should be used for the entire act of sex. Keep in mind; condoms aren't 100% effective when it comes to preventing pregnancy or disease. However, they are very effective if you use them the right way.
- Avoid sharing underclothing or towels.
- Bathe after and before you have sex.
- If you are okay with vaccination, you can get vaccines for a lot of STDs, specifically Hep B and HPV.
- Make sure you are tested for HIV.
- If you abuse alcohol or drugs, please seek help. It is more common for people who are under the influence to have unsafe sex.
- Lastly, abstaining from sex completely is the only 100% effective way to prevent STDs.

There was a time when it was believed that using a condom with nonoxynol-9 would prevent STDs by killing the organisms that caused them. There has been new research that has found that this can end up irritating the woman's cervix and vagina and could increase her risk of an STD. It is recommended that you avoid condoms with nonoxynol-9.

# HERBAL MEDICINE

Nature is a generous mother and gives her sons all the tools they need to thrive in harmony with each other.

## Agave

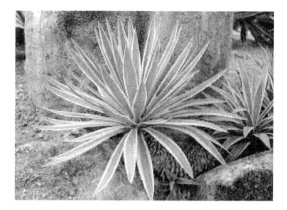

It possesses a low glycemic index which helps to keep blood sugar levels in check. This is one plant that is beneficial for boosting the immune system.

Medicinal Parts:

- The sap
- The leaves
- The seed

Influence on the Body:

- It helps improve metabolism
- It improves heart health
- It can help with depression
- Traditional Uses:
- Wound healing agent
- Hand skin treatment
- Soap production

## Alder

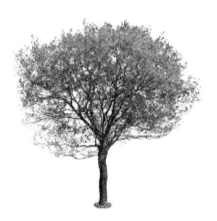

DR. SEBI BIBLE: 14 IN 1

Alder is a tree whose leaves and barks are used for making medicine. This medicine helps the body fight sore throats, rheumatism, swellings, and fever. Everyone can take alder, but individual dosing depends on age and severity of health condition. This is why people who take other medications need to be careful using alder.

Medicinal Parts:

- The bark
- The leaves

Influence on the Body:

- It helps to combat fever
- It reduces symptoms of constipation
- Traditional Uses:
- Bleeding

Possible Side Effects:

- None

## Alfalfa

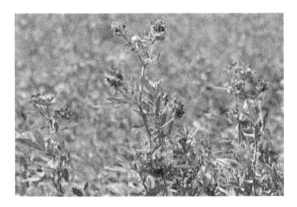

This herb has seeds, sprouts, and leaves adapted for medicinal use, mostly for kidney, bladder, and prostate conditions. It contains many essential nutrients, which makes it popular for constant use.

Medicinal Parts:

- The seeds
- The leaves

Influence on the Body:

- It helps improve metabolism
- It lowers cholesterol levels
- It contains healthy antioxidants
- Traditional Uses:
- Relieving menopause symptoms

## *Aloe Vera*

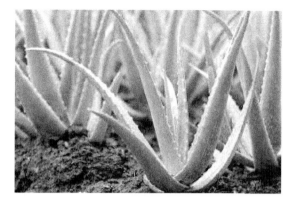

Parts to collect for medical purposes:

Leaves juice.

The poultice of fresh leaves was used to treat wounds, insect bites, and burns in general. A mostly unknown use of these fresh leaves poultice is that poultice was put into cheesecloth to dry. The dried poultice was then ground to obtain a fine powder used as a topical treatment for open wounds to stop bleeding and for blisters to absorb the moisture and avoid infections. If diluted into water, the powder was used to regulate the menstrual cycle or expel intestinal worms.

## *Amaranth*

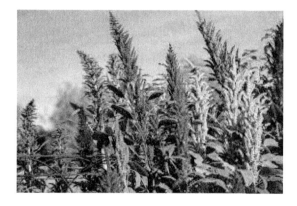

**Parts to collect for medical purposes:**

**Leaves**

**Flowers**

The decoction or raw consumption of leaves was used for its astringent characteristic and to reduce excessive menstruation (hypermenorrhea). The decoction of leaves was also used as gargling for throat inflammation.

Seeds were used as food for sustainment. You grinding them and prepare bread or cakes. Leaves (raw and cooked) and roots (boiled) are edible too.

*Angelica*

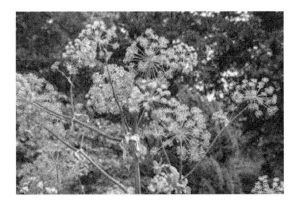

**Parts to collect for medical purposes:**

**Roots**

**Leaves**

**Flowers**

**Seeds**

The fresh root poultice on swollen joints or any kind of discoloration from mild to severe had an anti-inflammatory and pain relief effect on the part treated.

The decoction was the preferred way for Natives to extract the phytochemicals and use Angelica for healing purposes.

In detail, the decoction of leaves and flowers was used to cure all sorts of diseases: rheumatism, sore throats, fevers, ulcers, Urinary Tract Infections, and headaches. It was considered a panacea for every condition.

It is also a powerful carminative and helped with intestinal gas and a powerful anti-inflammation gargle in sore throat.

The raw consumption of leaves was used for its astringent characteristic to treat diarrhea. The same effect has been ascribed to the raw consumption of roots.

Seed decoctions were used to treat increase menstrual flow, in the case of hypermenorrhea.

In my opinion, the handiest way for Angelica assumption is by tinctures: the tincture of roots (dosage: 40 drops, three to four times a day) or seeds (dosage: 20 drops, three to four times a day) is beneficial in treating the condition listed above in a timesaving manner.

Other uses of Angelica in the Native American culture, besides the medical purpose, are related to religion (dried leaves and flowers were used to be smoked in the sacred pipe ceremony).

In addition, seeds were used as food for sustainment. You can create flour by grinding them and prepare bread or cakes, in many South American typical dishes. Leaves (raw and cooked) and roots (boiled) are edible too.

## Arsemart

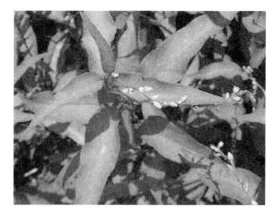

Parts to collect for medical purposes:

Whole plant.

Poultice and juice of the herb were used on ulcers and swollen joints, both topically and internal due to its mild analgesic characteristics. For the same reason, the chewing of the root was used to treat toothache.

One of the most common uses was related to the treatment of parasite worms: the tea obtained from leaves and flowers is effective in the case of sepsis and intestinal worms. The recommended dosage is 1 tsp. of the dried herb infused in 1 cup of boiling water for half an hour; the infusion must be drunk throughout the day two or three tablespoonfuls at the time. The topical application of drops of diluted tincture inside the ear was used to kill worms within.

## Arnica

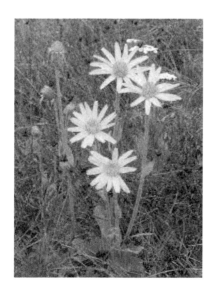

Arnica is an herb that is commonly used for treating bruises, and the leaves are also used to treat certain muscle-related conditions. It usually was administered orally and is applied in a gel-like manner. It has often been taken topically to help prevent overdosing on the drug.

The best way to take arnica is through homeopathic solutions. Let it dissolve slowly until it is completely diluted before ingesting it. It is bad for health to take the plant directly as it is.

Arnica is useful for pain management, and compared to other drugs; people do not get addicted to it.

**Medicinal Parts:**

**The flower**

**The leaves**

**Influence on the Body:**

**It helps to reduce inflammation**

**It helps bring down joint pains and swellings**

**Traditional Uses:**

**Aches and pain relief**

**A cure for bruises**

*Ashwagandha (Indian Ginseng)*

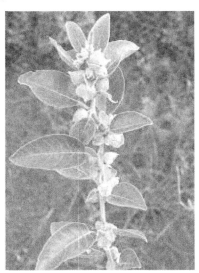

Parts to collect for medical purposes:

- Root (dried).

Herbal Medicine Use: The tea obtained by mixing 1 tsp of powdered root in 1 cup of boiling water is effective in stomachache and indigestion. Another effect of it is related to the treatment of stress and anxiety. The recommended use of the above tea is one cup maximum, drunk three or four times throughout the day. Another use of the Ashwagandha is related to the poultice obtained from pounding the fresh leaves. This can be used as an antibiotic and anti-inflammatory remedy for topical application on wounds.

*Aspen*

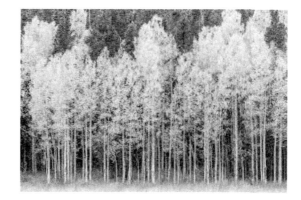

The bark and aspen leaves also have medicinal purposes like treating joint, nerve, and bladder challenges. It contains chemicals similar to what is found in aspirin, known as salicin, and this is known to help reduce inflammation.

Medicinal Parts:

- The bark
- The leaves

Influence on the Body:

- It helps treat rheumatoid arthritis
- It helps to manage nerve pain
- It helps treat swellings that come from infections

*Balsam Fir*

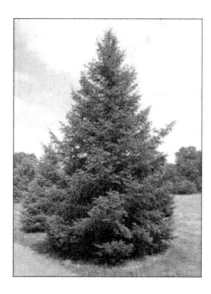

Parts to collect for medical purposes:

Sap

Roots

Barks

Leaves

Main effect: Analgesic and Antiseptic.

The decoction of barks was used to reduce fever and stimulate sweating to detoxify the body. Also, needle tea was used to cure respiratory problems and colds due to its astringent characteristics.

Finally, the sap is used directly to treat burns and close wounds. Raw consumption of it is used to prevent colds and sore throats.

Minor use of this balsamic sap was during the sweat lodge ceremony: the sap was dripped on the hot stones to create aromatic steam.

*Black Haw*

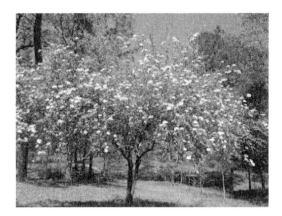

Parts to collect for medical purposes:

- Barks
- Root
- Main effect: Diuretic, Astringent, Nervine, Antispasmodic.

Native American healers used Black Haw root bark decoction to prevent miscarriages in women. The prescription was to take the root bark decoction three weeks before the last miscarriage happened and continue for three weeks after. If no miscarriage of other uterus contractions happened after the three weeks, the cure could be stopped.

The benefits of the root bark decoction did not limit the prevention of miscarriages: it is known for its use as a powerful febrifuge and in case of diarrhea when other treatments failed.

*Blueberry*

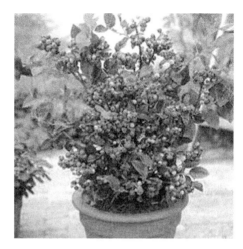

Parts to collect for medical purposes:

- Leaves
- Berries.

Main effect: Diuretic, Astringent.

Natives used to prepare tea from dried leaves as a remedy for diarrhea and used this drink as a topical wash for skin conditions like dermatitis and rashes of all sort.

An interesting application of this shrub was the consumption of the powder of dried leaves to reduce the sensation of nausea immediately.

Besides the obvious raw consumption, a simple preparation you can make regarding the fruits. In the comfort of your kitchen is the alcohol infusion to treat spasmodic diarrhea and Irritable Bowel Syndrome. The instructions are quite simple: place dried blueberry in a glass bottle and cover it with 95% Alcohol. Let the bottle rest for at least one month in a shaded place. The recommended dosage for this remedy is 1 tbsp. of the alcoholic infusion in four oz. of distilled water.

*Black Locust*

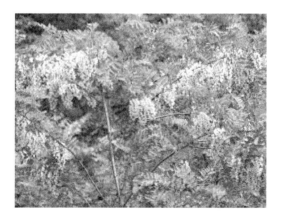

The black locust is a medium-sized melliferous tree found in North America. Native Americans have used the dried leaves of the black locust for treating burns and wounds. It can likewise be used to treat internal conditions like stomach burns and for individuals who have stomach conditions.

It simply helps with digestion and covers some of the digestion-related complications. It also has sedating and calming effects on the body, and this is great for adults and children who have insomnia and overall difficulty falling asleep.

Medicinal Parts:

- The leaves
- The flowers
- The fruit

Influence on the Body:

- It helps to improve the digestion
- Pain reliever
- Easing digestion

*Black Walnut*

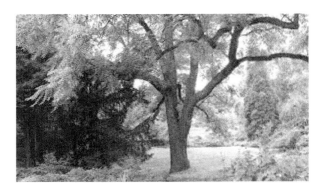

Compared to the usual nuts we know; the black walnut is not grown in orchards, and it grows in most Native American locations. It is rich in protein and contains many other vitamins, minerals, and fiber. It contains many antioxidants that make the body healthy, preventing some of the worst complications to the immune system, like diabetes and cancer.

The great thing about this is that it can easily be incorporated into the diet by adding it to other dishes for tasty and healthy diets.

Medicinal Parts:

- The nut

**Influence on the Body:**

**Reduces risks of diabetes, cancer, and even heart complications**

**Beauty and radiance support**

**Digestive support**

*Bloodroot*

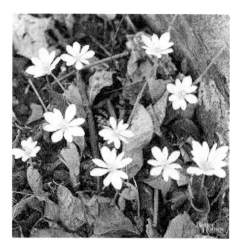

Bloodroot is a helpful plant, and people use the underground stem to make medications. The medications made from the bloodroot are used to empty the bowel and cause people to vomit anything bad which has been ingested. It is versatile, helping you treat other challenges like sore throats, muscle and joint pains, and fever.

It is also used topically around wounds and cuts to improve healing properties and remove all the dead tissue from the affected area. In the early 1800s, bloodroot extracts were applied to the chests worn to help treat their breast tumors and other breast-related complications.

This was not all; bloodroot was applied to the tooth to prevent plaque buildup. This leaves the tooth and the gums healthy and protected from any tooth-related diseases.

Medicinal Parts:

- The underground rhizome

Influence on the Body:

- It helps to cause vomiting and emptying of the bowels
- It helps with the treatment of sore throats
- Treatment of fever

## Blue Cohosh

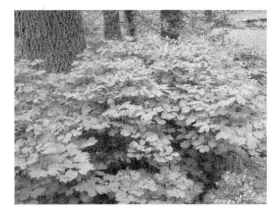

The blue cohosh is a plant with a name derived from the Indian word Algonquin meaning "rough," and it points to the representation of the root, which is rough. This root is used for making medicine, but it is not safe on its own. However, it is still available for use as a far better and safer medication than direct ingestion.

One of the major things with black cohosh is that it stimulates the uterus and makes it easy for women in labor to put to bed. It likewise helps calm menstruating women preventing some of the pains of menstruation, like muscle spasms.

It also helps to treat certain internal complications related to the infection of the internal organs and joints. The seed of the black cohosh can be roasted and taken as a drink, which is a much-preferred and healthy substitute to coffee.

**Medicinal Parts:**

**Influence on the Body:**

**Sore throat treatments**

**Treating uterus infections**

*Blue Spruce*

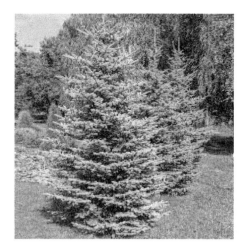

This evergreen tree has its genus name derived from pix, which means sticky resin. There are numerous benefits of using blue spruce, and they range from treating lung challenges, colds, throat problems, and measles.

Medicinal Parts:

- The cones
- The central portion
- The inner bark

Influence on the Body:

- It helps reduce tension and stress in the muscles
- It brings emotional balance
- It helps to tackle lung challenges
- Teas and salves for cold
- Poultice on rheumatic joints, on the chest and the stomach to relieve congestion and pain

*Boneset*

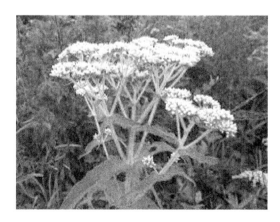

Parts to collect for medical purposes:

- Leaves
- Flowers
- Main effect: Febrifuge, Diaphoretic, Carminative.

Native Americans used boneset leaves and flowers in many medical preparations. For example, the tea obtained from the infusion of dried leaves was considered a powerful febrifuge. It was also used to treat most severe diseases such as malaria, pneumonia, arthritis, and gout.

Talking about gout and arthritis it is important to report also the topical application of the poultice obtained by pounding fresh leaves and flowers, as a topical anti-inflammatory treatment on swollen joints and other contusive traumas to the joints.

The double infusion of the roots was used as an emetic in food poisoning and to cure sore throat with gargling.

*Borage*

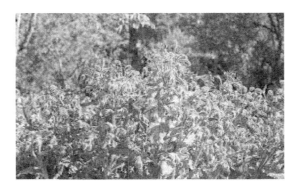

The borage is a plant with seed oils, flowers, and leaves used for numerous medical purposes. This plant can easily be grown in your gardens, and it can likewise be commercially cultivated to extract the borage seed oil. This plant also contains alkaloids that are carcinogenic and healthy.

The oil derived from the borage seeds treats skin disorders like rashes, eczema, and other topical skin conditions. It can also be used for other inflammation-related internal conditions like pains and swellings. Likewise, it is added to infant formulas for added fatty acids, which are required for the development of preterm infants. Hormonal problems

The leaves and the flowers help with cough and even hormonal problems, which help to purify the blood. It can be eaten in salads and other tasty meals to get the best of the herb.

Medicinal Parts:

- The flower
- The leaves
- The seeds
- Influence on the Body:
- Preventing inflammation
- Treats coughs and fevers
- It helps to dress and soften the skin

## Buckthorn

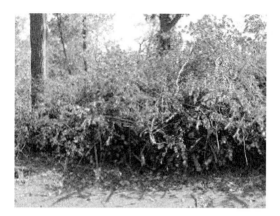

Buckthorn contains Vitamins, minerals, and amino acids that are useful for healthy living. The buckthorn's leaves, flowers, seeds, and berries make oils and teas healthy for many medical complications. It has antioxidant properties, which help cleanse the body and remove any free radicals in the blood.

This helps treat intestinal problems, regulate overall blood pressure, and prevent any heart challenges meaning improved immune functions. It is also applied topically as sunscreen or as a cosmetic for keeping the skin healthy.

Medicinal Parts:

- The leaves
- The flowers
- The berries
- The seed

Influence on the Body:

- Combats stomach upsets
- Prevents heart diseases
- Improves blood cholesterol
- Treats obesity
- Improves dry eyesight

*Burdocks*

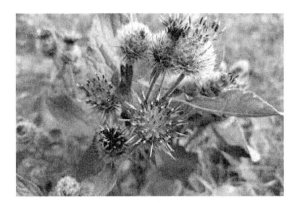

Burdock is a weed-covered in spores that can grow up to 4 feet tall. It is a genus plant that is part of the daisy flower, and it holds a lot of health benefits.

This plant is native to North America but is found in various world locations. The burdock plant's root, leaves, and seeds are used as medicine, but the root is sometimes consumed. It works as medicine because of the availability of chemicals that have high activities against inflammation and bacteria.

Medicinal Parts:

- The leaves
- The flowers
- The stalks
- The roots

Influence on the Body:

- It is used in the treatment of colds
- It helps to soothe joint pains
- It helps to treat skin conditions like psoriasis
- It helps to reduce syphilis

*Catnip*

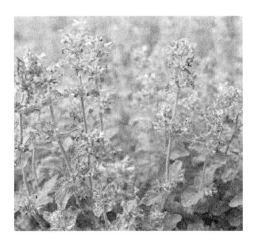

Parts to collect for medical purposes:

Leaves

Stems

Flowers

Native Americans used the infusion of the whole plant (leaves, stems, and flowers) for intestinal problems. The tonic effect of the plant reduces intestinal spasms and soothes inflammation related to diarrhea and dysentery. The infusion above also has a carminative effect, helping treat intestinal gas, and it was particularly indicated to calm menstrual cramps and dysmenorrhea.

Another use of the tea was related to its diaphoretic character: increased sweating would help in reducing fever states and in promoting overall detoxification of the body.

Another use of the plant was the topical application of the catnip poultice on swollen joints for pain relief in gout and rheumatism.

## Cattail

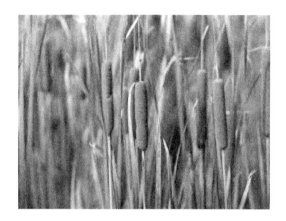

**Parts to collect for medical purposes:**

**Roots**

**Leaves**

Native Americans widely used the decoction of roots as a topical treatment for sunburns due to its emollient characteristics. Also, the flowers were used to treat wounds because they stop the bleeding and absorb excessive moisture. In addition, ashes obtained by burning leaves are antiseptic and were used to seal wounds and burns.

Besides the medical application of the plant, natives used it as food: in detail, roots were dried and grinder to obtain flour for bread and porridge, while hearts were boiled and eaten as vegetables.

## Chamomile

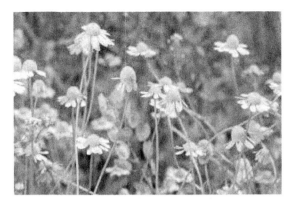

Parts to collect for medical purposes:

Flower

The fresh or dried plant infusion was used to soothe stomachache and cure excessive intestinal gas. Not only that, but the infusion was effective also on menstrual cramps, dysmenorrhea, and, if topically applied, to relieve skin inflammations, acne, and eczema.

The tea was also used as a tonic for nerves and calm anxiety and panic attacks. The mild soothing effect of this decoction was also used to treat arthritis and swollen joints pain.

A seemingly unknown use for this wonderful plant is related to meat preservation. The dried and powdered herb was on meat to absorb moisture and prevent it from rotting.

## Chaparral

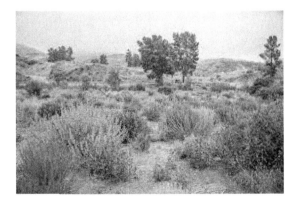

Chaparral has antioxidants and is used for curing several diseases like the common cold, tuberculosis, and even skin conditions. However, there needs to be proper regulation when it comes to dosage because if it is not taken the right way, it can lead to disorders in the liver, which people need to avoid at all costs.

Medicinal Parts:

- The leaves

Influence on the Body:

- Tuberculosis
- Common cold
- Complicated skin conditions
- Stomach pains
- Snakebite pains

*Chicory*

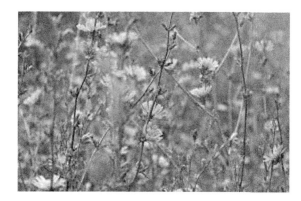

Chicory is a root fiber from a bright blue flower from the dandelion family. Native to North America and enjoyed for many years now, this root fiber is known for its medicinal properties and common use as a coffee alternative. The root has fiber extracted for use as a supplement or a food additive.

It contains insulin that inspires healthy gut bacteria growth, relieves constipation, increases stool frequency, and likewise helps to improve blood sugar control. One of the major things that was used back in the days was weight loss, as it helped curb the intake of calories and reduce appetite.

Medicinal Parts:

- The root
- The leaves

Influence on the Body:

- Stomach upsets
- Constipation
- Gall bladder disorders
- Traditional Uses:
- It was traditionally used for treating cuts, bruises, and sinus problems

*Cranberry*

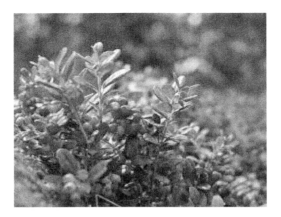

**Parts to collect for medical purposes:**

**Bark**

**Fruits**

The Natives used the medical properties of cranberries in the treatment of Urinary Tract Infections. This use is still actual nowadays in the case of cystitis and kidney stones.

To absolve to the purpose the berries were consumed raw, juiced, or, if only available in dried condition, as a tea. The cranberries have been scientifically proven to low the urine pH, thus promoting the dissolution of the sodium accumulations known as kidney stones and reducing the growth of bacterial infection in it that could cause UTIs.

The tea obtained with barks instead of dried berries, was extremely effective in treating menstrual pain and dysmenorrhea and was used also as a topical wash for infected wounds and skin ulcers because, due to its astringent properties, it promoted the formation of scarring tissue.

*Dandelion*

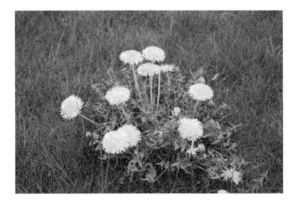

Parts to collect for medical purposes:

- Roots

Besides the raw consumption of the leaves for food, Native Americans used dandelion also for its medical properties.

Root decoction was used for cleansing and detoxification in liver and gallbladder conditions because it helped digestion and had a laxative effect. The diuretic properties of the decoction were widely known and the antispasmodic properties of the dandelion were also used to treat menstrual cramps and Pre-Menstrual Syndrome.

Root decoction was also used to increase lactation and stimulate the appetite via the promotion of bile production.

Finally, it is scientifically proved that dandelion raw consumption of leaves reduces the cholesterol level in the blood flow. This is because reduces the cholesterol absorption from food.

*Devil's Club*

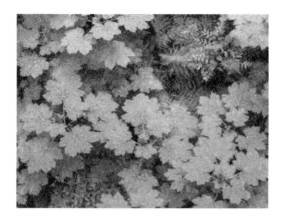

Parts to collect for medical purposes:

- Root
- Barks

Natives used this plant for ceremonial and sacred purposes. The root bark decoction was used as a tonic for nerves due to its qualities similar to ginseng. Other than that, the plant was used as a dye for tissues and as a traditional body painting for warriors (ashes of the burnt devil's club were mixed to grease to create the paint that was said to protect during battle).

*Echinacea*

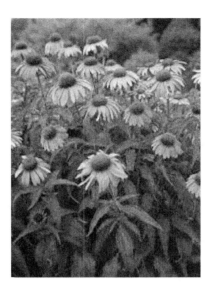

**Parts to collect for medical purposes:**

**Flower**

**Leaves**

**Roots**

The medical properties of Echinacea are widely known all over the world. Ancient Greeks and Egyptians used this plant as a panacea for every disease since the dawn of time. Also, Native Americans were aware of its power and used it to treat many conditions.

Root decoction was used as an analgesic for sore throat, toothache, and stomach pain. The diaphoretic properties of the Echinacea were used to induce sweat, thus cleansing the body and reduce fever.

The poultice obtained by pounding flowers and leaves is used to treat wounds, acne, and many skin conditions. Also, the raw leaves' consumption helps fight microbial and fungal infection (such as candida) and has been proven to be a good antiviral.

*Elderberry*

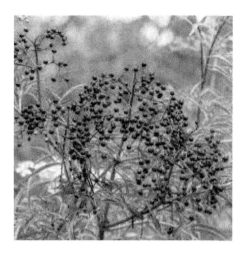

**Parts to collect for medical purposes:**

**The whole plant, from root to flowers and fruits**

Native Americans used to prepare tea with flowers to reduce fever and stimulate diuresis. This tea was also used in topical application in case of itching or painful skin conditions such as urticaria or rash.

The above tea was indicated for many respiratory system problems, from mild to severe: it was a treatment for asthma, allergies, sinusitis, and bronchitis.

The bark decoction had different effects, promoting bowel movement for a laxative action.

Finally, the mild toxicity of the berries was used to create a powerful analgesic by preparing a decoction of the berries, which soothed back pain, menstrual cramps, and rheumatisms.

*Feverfew*

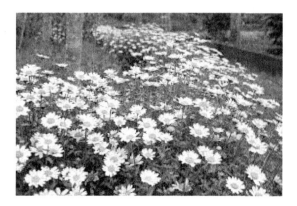

Parts to collect for medical purposes:

- Flower

As the name suggests, Natives used this plant to help in reducing the fever. The tea obtained from the flower is a powerful febrifuge used to treat headaches due to its mild sedative action.

*Geranium*

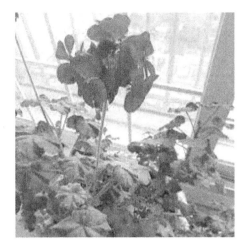

Parts to collect for medical purposes:

- Leaves
- Flowers
- Roots

A widely unknown use of the geranium is emergency medication in case of injuries. It is a powerful anti-hemorrhagic and the whole plant (leaves, flowers, and roots) was pounded in poultice directly on deep wounds to stop the bleeding. Usually, the plant was chewed to create the poultice and add to the astringent and anti-hemorrhagic action, the antiseptic action of the saliva.

Root was used in poultice and decocted: poultice was instead used to treat hemorrhoids, while root decoction was used for toothache.

*Goldenseal*

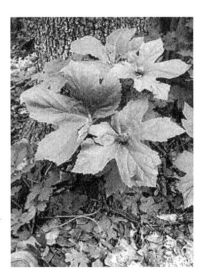

Parts to collect for medical purposes:

- Rhizome

Native Americans used the decoction of dried rhizomes and roots to treat dysentery due to its specific astringent characteristics. This decoction was also used for its emollient and anti-inflammatory properties as a wash for skin inflammation or conjunctivitis. The raw consumption of the root was indicated to benefit from these characteristics in the treatment of cough and sore throat.

The root extraction was widely used for curing scrofula and as a panacea for every liver and gallbladder condition.

The powdered dried rhizome was applied on wounds and burns to prevent infections due to its antiseptic properties. Also, is was considered a powerful anti-fungal.

WARNING: The consumption of this herb is not allowed during pregnancy or lactation. In addition, excessive consumption may result in food poisoning.

*Gooseberry*

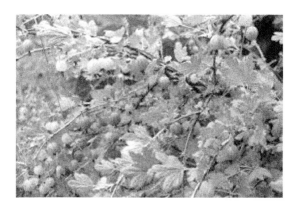

Parts to collect for medical purposes:

- Fruits
- Roots

Besides the raw consumption of fruits, Native Americans used the plant for medical purposes. The tea obtained by the dried fruits was gargles to soothe sore throats.

Also, the decoction of roots was used as a wash for eye inflammation or drunk directly, due to its vermifuge characteristics, to treat intestinal worms. Finally, the poultice of fruits and leaves was used to cure skin inflammation due to its emollient feature. It was believed that it cured snakebites because snakes were frightened by the plant.

*Hawthorn*

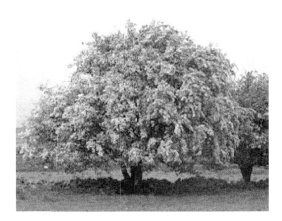

**Parts to collect for medical purposes:**

**Leaves**

**Fruits**

The Natives used hawthorn leaves to treat minor wounds when no other treatment was available. Leaves were simply chewed and the poultice applied on wounds and burns for easy emergency medication.

The plant was also used to prepare a decoction from seeds, that was used to treat diarrhea. The said decoction was also used as a mild sedative, mostly in heart palpitation.

The medical use of this plant was always associated with heart diseases by Native Americans and surprisingly by many other ancient populations all over the globe. In time, recent studies have proved that it has a positive effect on the main heart disease as tachycardia and hypertension and may help lower cholesterol levels.

*Hop*

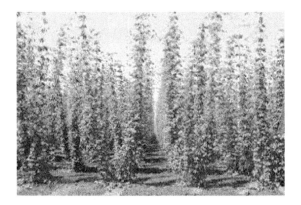

Hop has a mixed history as they are cultivated in many regions around the globe. Hebrews used hopes to fight the plague. At the same time, several Native American tribes independently discovered their healing proprieties as a sedative, toothache relief, and digestive aid. By the 1900s, the hop was already well-known in the United States and widely used in medicine. Meanwhile, Europeans used it as a preservative and flavoring agent in the beer brewing process.

Medicinal Parts:

- The cones
- The strobes

Influence on the Body:

The dry flower helps with anxiety and insomnia, restlessness, tension, excitability, nervousness, and irritability

The extracts of hop cones are used as a gentle tranquilizer and bitter stomachic

Hop extract also help with skin conditions and as an oil-free moisturizer

Hop is excellent to improve rosacea condition as they reduce heat in the skin and redness

- Sedative and digestive tonic
- The female inflorescences of the hop plant are used in brewing for their antibacterial effect and to add bitterness and aroma to beers

*Horsetail*

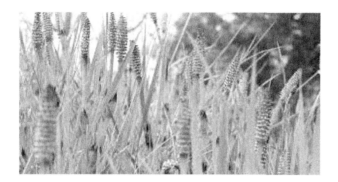

Parts to collect for medical purposes:

- Leaves
- Roots

Native Americans used this plant for medical purposes for both humans and horses. It is interesting to recall its use to create a decoction to treat the cough of horses.

The main medical purpose for humans was instead related to its diuretic qualities: the tea obtained with the needle-like branches was used to treat painful urination in case of Sexual Transmitted Disease and Urinary Tract Infections in general. Also, the bath obtained by infusing the branches in hot water was used to treat gonorrhea and syphilis.

The stem, reduced to a poultice, is used in topical applications for skin rash.

*Horsemint*

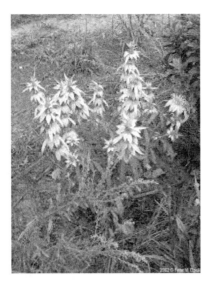

Horsemint is a bitter plant that tastes and smells like thyme. It has many medicinal properties, so it can combat numerous digestive problems, with gas being a major concern.

Traditionally, women take horsemint to help them enjoy their periods and tackle painful periods. Horsemint is not used by pregnant and nursing mothers to prevent unwanted reactions with the baby.

Medicinal Parts:

- The leaves
- The stem

Influence on the Body:

- It helps to treat digestive problems
- It helps to treat painful periods
- Traditionally used for treating diarrhea, stomach problems, and nausea

*Hyssop (New Mexico Giant)*

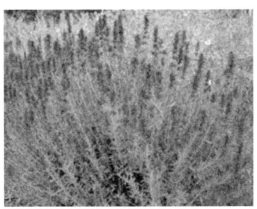

Parts to collect for medical purposes:

- The whole plant.

The salves and oils obtained by the whole plant were used to treat cough, by dissolving it in boiling water and inhaling the steam. The oil extraction plan's recommended preparation is to powder the dried plant into a mortar and then transfer it into a glass dish. The powder is then submerged in the oil of your choice (olive, canola, etc...) and cooked overnight in your kitchen oven at low temperature (170°F). The oil extraction is then obtained by straining the mixture using a cheesecloth. The oil is then gently heated on a stove and thickened with beeswax to obtain the salve.

Another use of the hyssop is preparing tea from the whole plant to reduce fever. Finally, dried and powdered leaves were used topically on wounds and sores.

*Juniper*

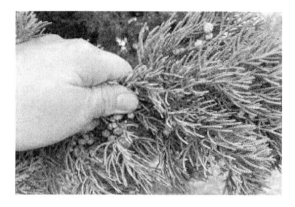

Parts to collect for medical purposes:

- Berries

Besides the widely documented application of the dried berries as a spice for game meat, this plant was also widely used for its medical purposes, not only by natives but also by Mediterranean cultures.

For example, the decoction obtained from the berries can help in premenstrual syndrome and dysmenorrhea. Also, it was used for its diuretic and antiseptic properties to treat Urinary Tract Infections and gallbladder conditions. Needles and bark could be added to the decoction to enhance the effect.

*Lady's Slipper*

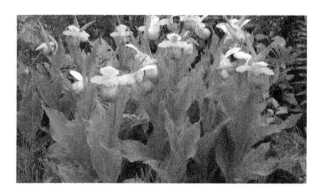

Lady's slipper is useful for treating anxiety-related conditions, emotional tension, and even insomnia. For children, Lady's slippers can be used to reduce their hyperactivity. Adults can also apply it topically to relieve cramps, twitches, and muscle spasms. This root is beneficial when used, but it can have reactions like allergic reactions for sensitive and restless people. It is not great for pregnant women.

**Medicinal Parts:**

**The root**

**Influence on the Body:**

**Insomnia**

**Anxiety**

**Nervous tension**

**It was traditionally used for tooth pains and muscle spasms**

*Lemon Balm*

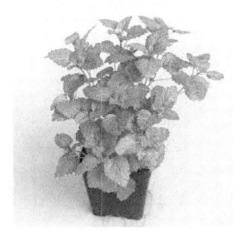

Parts to collect for medical purposes:
- Leaves
- Flowers
- Stems

Native Americans used the tea prepared with the aerial parts of the plant for its many benefits. The carminative qualities of lemon balm helped with intestinal gas. Moreover, its analgesic effect was used to calm nerves and, in combination with the anticonvulsant substances contained in it, helped treat menstrual cramps. Finally, the diaphoretic substances inside it induce sweat and promote cleansing of the body and a lowering of body temperature in case of excessive fever.

This plant is perfect for the black thumbs because it is infesting and rather inextirpable. It covers all the ground so its cultivation is advised in pots inside your home. The traditional harvesting period of lemon balm is spring for leaves and summer for flowers.

## Licorice (Wild American)

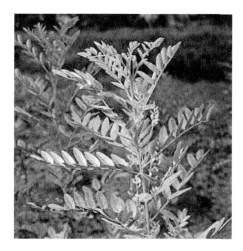

Parts to collect for medical purposes:

- Roots (dried)
- Leaves

Native Americans widely used the licorice for medical purposes, mainly related to stomach conditions. The decoction prepared with the peeled, dried root was used for laxative purposes in constipation. Another use of this tea was to reduce the fever because the diaphoretic substances induced sweat on the patient.

Other medical uses of the wild licorice were related to the tea of leaves, used as a topical medicament for earache, and the raw root consumption for toothache and sore throat.

Finally, the poultice obtained from the fresh root was used topically on swollen joints in case of rheumatism or gout.

## Maple

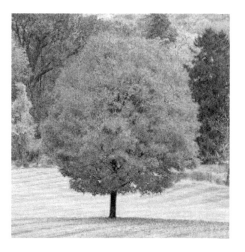

Parts to collect for medical purposes:

- Inner bark
- Leaves

Native Americans widely used the maple in their day-to-day lives. Its sap was the best source of sugar available for them. They collected it during winter and spring and used it as a sweetener. The same process is done today to harvest and produce maple syrup.

Besides the sustenance, maple was also used for its healing properties: the leaves infusion was used for detoxification, while the inner bark decoction was used as a wash for conjunctivitis and other eye conditions. If drunk, the inner bark decoction has an expectorant effect helping remove the phlegm in case of cough and sore throat.

## *Milkweed*

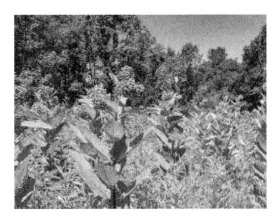

**Parts to collect for medical purposes:**

**Flowers**

**Leaves**

**Roots**

Native Americans used milkweed flowers only after accurate preparation due to their high toxic substances (cardiac glycosides). They were used as food, after boiling them. Seeds were crushed to obtain flour to prepare bread.

The medical applications of this plant are many. From the decoction of the dried roots used to increase lactation to the topical application of sap from leaves, to treat warts, urticaria, and insect bites.

Also, the poultice of leaves was used to treat wounds and the dried leaves infusion was used to treat stomach problems.

## Mullein

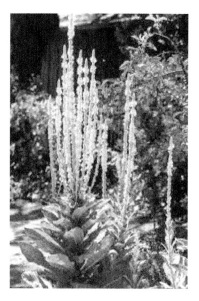

Parts to collect for medical purposes:

- Flowers
- Leaves

The demulcent effect of the mullein (leaves and flowers) were widely known by Native Americans who used it in decoction and teas to treat mild respiratory conditions, from cough to nasal congestion.

The action of mullein was frequently paired with the one of other plants like thyme and rosemary.

The poultice obtained from fresh leaves was used to treat wounds, swellings, and skin ailments such as rashes, while dried ones were smoked to induce cough and expectorate the phlegm.

## Mint

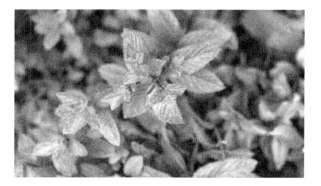

Mint grows in wet environments and moist soils, and it can reach a height of 4-45 inches tall and spread across a big expanse of land. Consuming mint has many health benefits, such as improving irritable bowel syndrome, relief from digestive problems, and improved brain functions.

Medicinal Parts:

- The leaves
- The flower
- The stem
- The bark
- The seeds

Influence on the Body:

- It helps to relieve indigestion
- It helps to improve brain functions
- It reduces breastfeeding pains
- Traditionally used for treating irritable bowel syndrome

## Nettle

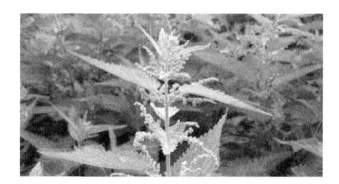

Parts to collect for medical purposes:

Roots

Leaves

Native Americans widely used the nettle to treat many conditions related to the upper respiratory tract. It is widely documented that the infusion of fresh leaves and stems is used to treat allergies, cough, or even asthmatic conditions.

One of the most effective treatments you can do in the comfort of your kitchen using nettle is the tincture of fresh nettle by using a weight ratio between herb and 50% Alcohol solution of 1:2. By simply soaking fresh nettle leaves in the alcoholic solution for 2 weeks in a shadowy place, and straining the liquid, you will have access to a powerful preventive treatment in case of bronchitis, flu, and colds in general. Just assuming 20 drops of the tincture two times a day (I prefer to do it first thing in the morning and just before dinner), in the proximity of the cold season will shield you from the possibility to catch a cold or flu.

Native Americans also used the dried and powdered plant on wounds and burns in topical application to stop bleeding and as a disinfectant. The dried leaves were also used to prepare a diuretic tea recommended in Urinary Tract Infections.

A curious application of nettle was for pain relief in case of swollen joints due to arthritis or gout:

fresh, stinging stems were beaten on the swollen joints to create a counter-inflammation that would recall blood and relieve some of the pain due to the swelling.

*Oat*

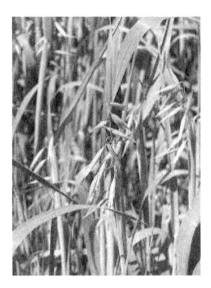

Popular and widely distributed in most parts of the world today, oats are a commercially flaked grain known as oatmeal. The tincture and powder are used in herbal tonics and capsules.

It is a recognized natural food with an appealing taste to help patients with weak digestive systems. The tincture is used as a neutralizer for the sexual gland system. It also helps to restore the body after a stressful event.

Medicinal Parts:

- The straw
- The seeds

Influence on the Body:

- Fever
- Indigestion
- Exhaustion
- It was traditionally used as decoration, tea, and for treating fever
- It was also used as cosmetic aid to improve skin outlook

## Oregon Grape

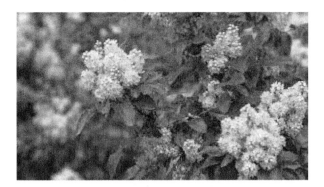

Medicinal Parts

Roots

Native Americans used Oregon Grape in many ways. Above all, fruits were renowned to induce vomit if eaten in small quantities.

The decoction of stems was used to promote detoxification of the liver and gallbladder. Decoction of bark was used for the same purpose and as an eyewash for conjunctivitis or a gargle for tonsillitis.

Roots were used in decoctions to treat upset stomach due to Oregon Grape astringent properties and in extraction as a topical treatment on the skin for ulcers and excessive dryness.

## Passionflower

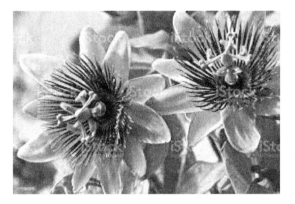

On colonization in Europe, this herb was mostly used for treating anxiety-related conditions, while the fruits were used as flavors in many delicious beverages. One of the significant reasons this flower is great for anxiety is its calming effect on the mind. It helps boost the level of gamma-aminobutyric acid (GABA) in your brain, which helps to calm the mind, helping you sleep better.

Medicinal Parts:

- The above-ground parts

Influence on the Body:

- It helps to relieve insomnia

- It helps to relieve anxiety
- It was traditionally used to treat seizures and anxiety

## Plantain

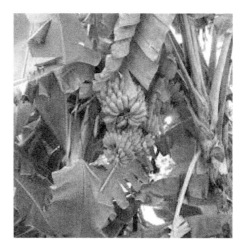

Medicinal Parts:

- The leaves
- The seeds

Influence on the Body:

- Diarrhea
- Yeast infection
- Cough
- Baby Rash
- Bee bites
- Eczema
- Dye for fabrics

## Red Clover

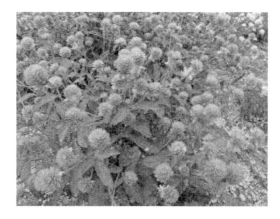

Parts to collect for medical purposes:

- Leaves
- Flowers

Native Americans used red clover tea as a tonic and for all the respiratory conditions from asthma to cough. In addition, this decoction was used as a wash for wounds and burns due to its astringent characteristics and as a remedy for menopausal side problems, particularly hot flashes. The diaphoretic effect of the tea helps in cleansing the body and regulates the thyroidal hormone production that causes the hot flash / chilling sensations.

## Sagebrush

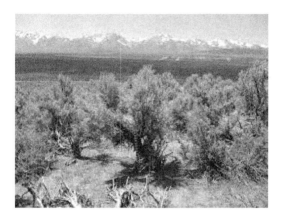

## Parts to collect for medical purposes:

### Leaves

Native Americans considered this plant sacred due to its scent with sage. They used the plant for the smudging ceremony and to chase demons away. In addition, it was used in the sweat lodge ceremony due to its aromatic properties.

The medical use of the plant mainly relies on the decoction of leaves. It was considered a powerful febrifuge because it induced sweat and promoted the lowering of body temperature. In addition, this decoction was used to help the uterus to contract in difficult childbirths and to treat stomachache.

If used as a gargle, the astringent properties of the decoction helped with sore throat and bronchitis. Moreover, this tea was used as a wash for the eyes in cases of conjunctivitis.

Finally, a small tent was created between a bowl containing the hot decoction of leaves and the patient's head, using a canvas or a pelt. The patient inhaled the steam of the decoction to benefit from the expectorant qualities of the aromatic substances of the sagebrush, to promote the excretion of phlegm and mucus from the upper respiratory tract.

The poultice of fresh leaves was applied over wounds and helped heal due to its antiseptic properties.

*Sassafras*

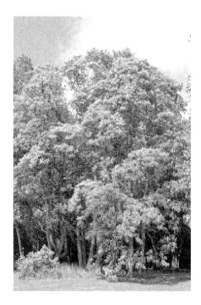

Parts to collect for medical purposes:

- Root
- Barks
- Leaves.

The Native Americans used the dried leaves as a spice, simply by powdering or roughly crushing them.

The decoction of roots was used as a tonic and for its detoxifying effects. Also, it will cause some relief to the symptoms of Sexual Transmitted Diseases such as syphilis or gonorrhea. The anticonvulsant effect of the root decoction was also an effective treatment for stomachache, menstrual pain, and cramps.

**Bark tea was instead used for its diaphoretic effects as a powerful febrifuge.**

*Saint John's Wort*

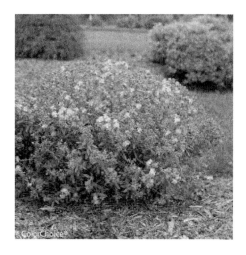

Parts to collect for medical purposes:

- The whole plant

Saint John's Wort is one of the most used officinal plants in herbal medicine worldwide. Native Americans were aware of its properties and widely used it in many preparations. It was considered a heal-all plant with astringent, anti-inflammatory, and antiseptic characteristics.

The whole plant decoction was used to treat menstrual problems, such as poor blood flow or Pre Menstrual Syndrome, for its emmenagogue properties. The stimulating effect on uterus contraction was also used to induce abortions and facilitate difficult childbirth.

Not only that, the tea obtained from flowers was used as a mild sedative to calm nerves and induce sleep in case of traumatic events or insomnia.

Regarding the fresh plant uses, we can mention the poultice of the whole plant was applied over wounds to facilitate healing and avoid infections due to its antiseptic properties. In addition, raw root consumption was used to treat snakebites. Finally, leaves and flowers were used raw as a buffer to treat wounds and nasal epistaxis because they immediately stopped bleeding.

## Sarsaparilla

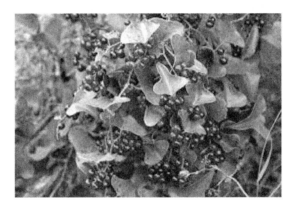

For many years, people used the root of the sarsaparilla plant for skin problems and the treatment of arthritis. It was later brought into European countries, where it was adopted for treating syphilis.

It contains phytochemicals with anti-inflammatory properties that help with joints and all types of body pains. It is healthy for those who have underlying medical conditions to consult their physician before taking any steps concerning usage.

Medicinal Parts:

- The roots

Influence on the Body:

- It is used for treating skin diseases
- It is used to increase urination and fluid retention
- It was traditionally used for treating leprosy and syphilis

## Seneca Snakeroot

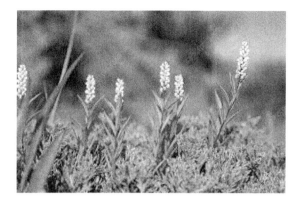

Seneca snakeroot is a plant with medicinal roots used by numerous individuals across the globe. It is used to manage inflammation and other health challenges like chest and throat infections, leading to asthma and emphysema. Traditionally the Seneca snakeroot was used by Native Americans for treating bites from the venomous rattlesnake.

It is also used for helping those who have difficulties sweating even when they exercise, clean the bowels, and clear sore throats. It is unsafe for direct consumption and can lead to nausea, vomiting, and dizziness.

Medicinal Parts:

- The spike
- The fruiting capsules
- The root

Influence on the Body:

- It is useful for treating the following:
- Asthma
- Chronic bronchitis
- Emphysema
- Chest inflammation
- It was traditionally used for treating pneumonia

## Skullcap

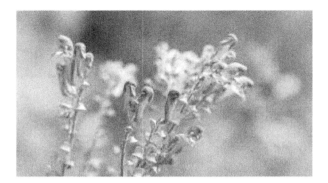

The skullcap has antioxidants and helps prevent and protect against neurological conditions like Parkinson's disease and depression. It is also scientifically proven to reduce the symptoms of an allergic reaction.

Adults can take the skullcap as tea, fluid extracts, tincture, or dried herbs for healthy consumption. On the other hand, children should not be given this herb no matter the circumstances. Even adults should take precautions when using it, mainly because it can react with specific supplements and drugs. Consult your trusted herbalist.

Medicinal Parts:

- The flower
- The leaves

Influence on the Body:

- It promotes relaxation
- It reduces your response to stress
- It supports healthy sleep patterns
- It was traditionally used as anxiety and tension therapy

## Slippery Elm

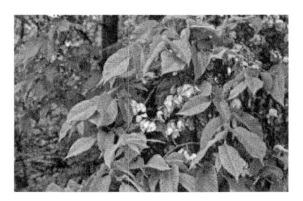

**Parts to collect for medical purposes:**

**Bark**

Native Americans widely used this indigenous elm species for medical purposes by preparing a decoction of the dried inner bark. The inner bark releases a mucilaginous substance that, if drunk, can help treat gastritis and ulcers by protecting the stomach walls; if used as a wash is a powerful emollient for wounds and burns. The same effects were obtained by the infusion of the powdered inner bark.

The outer bark decoction was used differently, to induce uterine contraction and causing abortions or helping difficult childbirths.

The salve obtained by thickening with beeswax the oil of outer bark is useful to treat colds, sore throat, and bronchitis by dissolving it in boiling water and inhaling the steam (fumigation).

*Sumac*

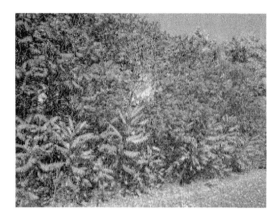

Parts to collect for medical purposes:

- Bark

Native Americans used the decoction of sumac bark as a wash to treat conjunctivitis and a gargle to treat sore throat. This decoction was also drunk to benefit from its astringent properties in dysentery and diarrhea.

The fresh leaves were pounded to create a poultice with anti-inflammatory properties to treat skin rash and urticarial with topical application.

*Tobacco*

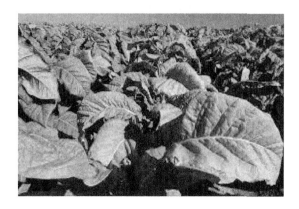

Parts to collect for medical purposes:

- Leaves
- Preferred Solvents: Water.
- Effects: Antispasmodic, Cathartic, Emetic, Analgesic.

Native Americans used tobacco mainly for ceremonial purposes, by smoking it in the sacred pipe. The plant was also used for some small medical purposes, for its analgesic properties. The poultice obtained by pounding the fresh leaves was used on joints swelling and scorpion stings to reduce the pain, and as a panacea for skin conditions. Fresh or powdered leaves were chewed to reduce headaches.

Finally, mixed with chalk, the leaves poultice was used as a primitive toothpaste to whiten the teeth.

## Valerian

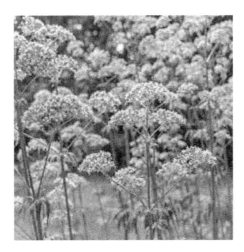

Parts to collect for medical purposes:

- Root

Valerian was widely known, not only among Native Americans but also among many ancient populations for its sedative action. The tea prepared from Valerian roots is a mild sedative and stress-relieving drink. It is sleep-inducing and so it is useful to treat insomnia. A side property of the root decoction is astringency, so this same decoction was also useful to treat diarrhea and colds.

The poultice of the roots can be used topically to treat wounds, burns, and skin inflammation in general.

The effect of this herb is enhanced when mixed with others, such as peppermint, gentian, and red clover.

## Venus's Slipper

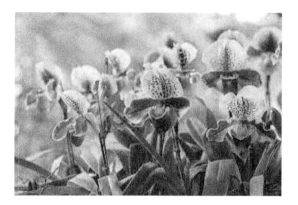

Parts to collect for medical purposes:

- Root

**The flower bulb was consumed raw or the flower sucked as a treatment for epilepsy.**

## Violet

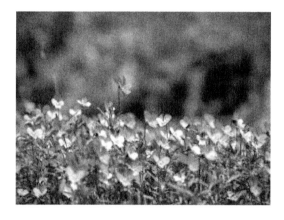

Parts to collect for medical purposes:

- Flowers
- Leaves

Native Americans used violet as a heal-all plant. The violet tea was used to regularize body function and reduce intestinal gas due to its carminative qualities. Also, it was considered effective in lowering the body temperature.

Gargling the infusion of dried flowers was indicated to reduce conditions related to throat inflammation and excessive mucus production such as sore throat, earaches, cough, and hoarseness.

## Verbena

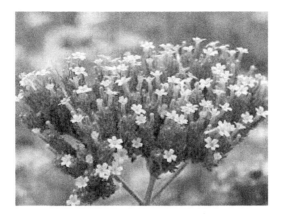

Verbena is a well-used herbal medicine used all over the globe for the treatment of numerous diseases. Its benefits include protecting the nerve cells, reducing convulsion, and preventing tumors. It also treats ear infections and can even be used as solar cream.

Verbena is used to stimulate and increase milk production while breastfeeding.

It is advisable to take verbena in processed forms such as powder, tea, or tincture.

Medicinal Parts:

- Parts above the ground

Influence on the Body:

- It is used for treating the following:
- Digestive disorders
- Trouble sleeping
- Agitation
- It was used for treating chest pains and related conditions

## Water Birch

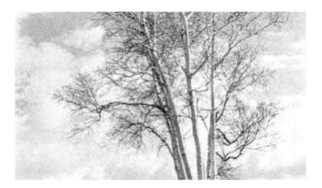

Parts to collect for medical purposes:

- Leaves
- Bark.

Native Americans used the Water Birch febrifuge properties by preparing a strong tea from leaves and barks. This drink could also be used to wash for mild skin ailments, such as pimples.

*Watercress*

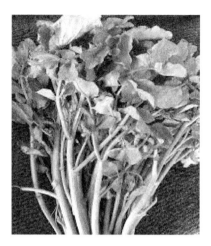

Parts to collect for medical purposes:

- Roots
- Leaves

The most documented use of this plant by Native Americans is leaves to spice their dishes due to their spicy and acrid taste.

The medical use is less known and indicates the raw consumption of the plant to treat cough, colds, and indigestion, due to its strong expectorant qualities. The astringent and expectorant properties of the plant will facilitate the removal of phlegm and excessive mucus in no time.

The plant has also strong diuretic characteristics and was indicated for cleansing and detoxifying.

*Wild Yam*

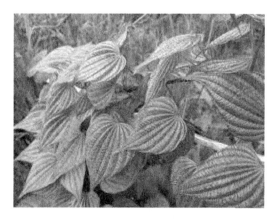

Wild Yam (Dioscorea Vilosa) is a tuberous species native to the eastern part of North America. While the wild yam is edible, the root is also helpful in treating hormonal conditions like menopause, and it is also useful for treating arthritis.

Wild yam is also helpful as an alternative to estrogen therapy, menstrual cram, premenstrual syndrome, weak bones, and male sex drive. Wild Yam creams are also helpful for topical application and can reduce hot flashes, a symptom of menopause.

Medicinal Parts:

- The entire tuber

Influence on the Body:

- It helps to treat the following conditions:
- Vaginal dryness in older women
- Menstrual cramps
- Osteoporosis
- It was used traditionally to increase the sexual drive and energy in men and increase women's breast size

## Willow

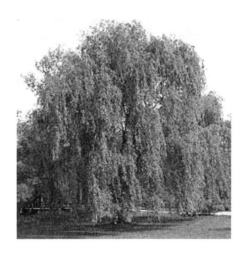

Parts to collect for medical purposes:

- Bark

Salix bark is rich in salicin, which is the natural molecule from which aspirin is derived. Natives and other ancient populations used Salix bark to treat colds, rheumatism, and headaches, using the febrifuge and analgesic properties of this plant.

Salix bark decoction was effective for pain relief in tendinitis, arthritis, and bursitis. Its anti-inflammatory properties helped reduce the swelling and the pain associated with those ailments.

## *Witch Hazel*

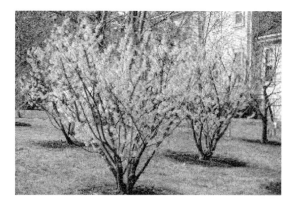

Witch Hazel (Hamamelis Virginiana) is a member of the witch hazel family. This shrub is native to North America and is used to produce ointments. These ointments are applied to the skin and scalp to help soothe sensitive skins as they prevent inflammation.

The witch hazel can be used as a natural treatment for inflammation, hemorrhoids, fighting acne, and soothing sore throats. This shrub is robust and fit for use without any health consequences. You just need to make sure that you take it in regulated quantities and not every time

Medicinal Parts:

- The twig
- The bark

Influence on the Body:

- Alleviates scalp sensitivity
- It helps treat hemorrhoids
- It fights acne
- Soothes sore throat
- Reduces skin irritation
- It was traditionally used for treating itchy and skin inflammations

## Yarrow

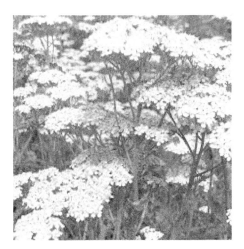

Parts to collect for medical purposes:

- Leaves
- Flowers
- Stem

Yarrow is one of the most used herbs in Native American medicine, mostly used in combination with others, such as passionflower or sage, to increase its effects.

A not-so-known, but widely adopted among Native Americans, usage of the plant is the snorting of dried and pulverized leaves to stop chronic epistaxis and headaches.

The poultice of leaves has a strong anti-inflammatory effect in mastitis, common skin ailments such as eczemas, or burns and wounds. Raw leaves can be used as an emergency medication if you hurt yourself in the woods, and if applied directly onto the wound they can immediately stop the bleeding.

Native Americans also used the tea obtained from the fresh plant to induce sweating and treat fever, inflammations, and infections. This decoction is also a strong diuretic and was considered depurative. This decoction was also used for its analgesic property as a topical wash in insect stings.

The infusion prepared with leaves only has a sedative effect and helps in relaxation and sleep, while the decoction of only roots was used as a wash for acne.

Tincture of yarrow effectively reduces excessive menstrual blood flow (hypermenorrhea).

Salves obtained from yarrow are effective if rubbed on the patient's chest in case of bronchitis.

Smudging of the dried plant keeps mosquitos away.

*Yellow Dock*

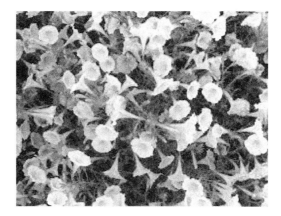

Parts to collect for medical purposes:

Rhizome

Native Americans used the anti-inflammatory properties to treat swollen joints and arthritis. A topical application of the poultice of fresh, mashed rhizome was indicated in these cases.

The juice of the rhizome or the roasted seeds features amazing astringent properties in treating diarrhea and dysentery.

The powder obtained by the dried rhizome was used as an anti-hemorrhagic on wounds.

The decoction of the dried rhizome, which is very bitter, is a powerful stimulant of the liver and helps detoxify the blood.

*Yucca*

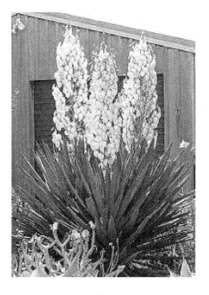

Parts to collect for medical purposes:

- Roots

- Leaves

Native Americans used this plant for hygienic purposes. Being rich in saponins, yucca roots extract was used as a natural soap to remove head lice.

The dried root decoction has been used to relieve gout and rheumatisms and is a powerful laxative. The water obtained by filtering the poultice of leaves is useful to calm uncontrolled vomit.

## Zizia Aurea (Golden Alexander)

Parts to collect for medical purposes:

- Flower
- Roots
- Leaves.

Native Americans used dried root powder as a powerful analgesic in teas and decoctions. The tea from leaves and flowers treats Pre Menstrual Syndrome and menstrual pain.

# HOW TO FOLLOW THE DIET

## Tips And Tricks For Following the Alkaline Diet Successfully

The primary mineral ingredients of earth, such as calcium, magnesium, titanium, zinc, and copper, reinforce the body. It is an alkaline diet to prevent asthma, malnutrition, fatigue, and even cancer. Is there something else capable of doing something like that? Here are ten tips for the successful implementation of the alkaline diet.

## Drink Water

Water is perhaps the most significant (after oxygen) resource for our body. As the water content influences, the chemistry of the body, hydration in the body is very important. To maintain the body well hydrated (filtered to cleaned), drink about 8-10 glasses of water.

## Stop Acidic Beverages Like Tea Coffee or Soda

Our body also seeks to control the content of acid and alkaline. In carbonated beverages, there is no need to blink, as the body rejects carbon dioxide as waste!

## Breathe

Oxygen is the reason our body functions, and if you provide the body with ample oxygen, it can function better. Sit down and enjoy deep breathing for two to five minutes. Nothing is simpler than being able to do yoga.

## Avoid Food with Preservatives and Food Colors

Our body has not been conditioned to consume these chemicals, and they are then absorbed or stored as fat by the body and do not affect the liver. Acids are formed by chemicals so that the body neutralizes them either by producing cholesterol or by blanching iron from the RBCs (leading to anemia) or by removing calcium from the bones (osteoporosis).

## Stop Artificial Sweeteners

These sweeteners are potentially toxic to the body and appear to be high in low fat. Saccharin, the main ingredient in sweeteners, also causes cancer. Therefore, stay away from these things. Go for more nutritious food, a good one at least.

## Exercise

They can also balance the alkaline element with the acidic element. This is not just a matter of alkaline milk intake. Natural bodywork is also influenced by a little acid (because of muscles).

Satiate Your Cravings by Eating Fruits or Soaked Nuts for a Snack

We still eat a little fast food while we are thirsty. Build a tradition of eating new vegetables or almonds, like walnuts.

Eat the Right Food Blend

When digested, the fats and proteins of carbohydrates require a particular environment. And don't eat all at once. Evaluate and correctly match the food composition to create the optimum mix of all the nutrients that you ingest.

Green Powders May Be Used as Replacements for Food

This helps to boost the body's alkaline consistency.

Even When Under Pressures Sleep Well Stay Calm and Composed

Strive to escape the pain. Our mind has control over the digestive system, and you can only know that it functions properly when in a calm, centered state. Relax, then, and stay safe.

## Alkaline Diet Plans

Many people are successful with their food plans, and implementing alkaline meal plans is the most important solution. As we can see, some people who have illnesses such as arthritis and cysts and people who have been obese and weak have been cured by this type of diet. Sickness is the greatest obstacle facing our lives. A person can't do things if he doesn't feel well; he or she might want to do it. He or she may not be able to do important things, so returns to an unhealthy lifestyle. The pH equilibrium must be maintained to function properly, and the normal pH of the body must be 7,365. Our body would, therefore, be alkaline rather than acidic. With our alkaline diet plans, there are many things we can remember to accomplish:

## Have the Best Understanding of What Alkaline Diet Is

What the alkaline diet means is fascinating to understand. We should note that an alkaline diet primarily consists of fresh fruits and vegetables that contain alkaline residues once metabolized in our bodies. Meats like beef, pork, and other refined foods, are not derived from alkaline food and must therefore be eaten in limited quantities.

## Plan for Your Meals Ahead of Time Ahead

Preliminary meal planning is a safe way to completely value and maintain effective eating habits. It is important that the foods that you need to prioritize are listed. Although it will take some time to do so, it will be helpful as you have sufficient opportunity to reflect and write down items that can contribute to a healthier lifestyle and improved consumption.

## Eat plenty of fruits and vegetables

Since alkaline foods are primarily fruits and vegetables, it is possible to eat more. These foods have negatively charged components that, when taken in by our bodies, neutralize the acids that are charged positively. The muscle, on the other hand, maintains a pH balance. Some acidic fruits and vegetables that are not recommended to be eaten in large amounts are also available.

## Know P.H. Balance's Value

We should be cautious about the types of food we consume if we know the importance of maintaining a pH balance. The fluids in our body must maintain a healthy degree of pH so that our cells continue to function properly. It does not mean, however, that we do ultimately not consume acidic foods. 75 percent-80 percent of alkaline and 20 percent-25 percent of acid products must be ingested to achieve a safe body state. It doesn't take so much time to change your life, but with the right under-standing, you can make significant changes in your lifestyle. With alkaline diet plans, we just need a balanced eating schedule. No one wants a sedentary life, so we've got to drive now.

# DR. SEBI SUPPLEMENTS

The very best approach to acquire the critical substances you desire (minerals, vitamins, essential fatty acids, fats—the list continues on and on) is via a balanced, healthful, nutritional supplement (one which is 100% natural if possible). However, the truth is that a number of individuals have quite a difficult time eating enough of the ideal sorts of foods to acquire the materials they require in the right amounts. That is why it is highly suggested that you carefully think about using nutritional sup-plements to improve the quantities of crucial stuff your body needs to have to work at its best.

It might appear overwhelming to consider carrying ten (or more) distinct supplements daily but re-member that doing this could be a true advantage to your body and head. Additionally, it might allow you to stay longer and much healthier. Nevertheless, if you are aware that you are getting a fantastic amount of a few of these chemicals in your diet plan and you are interested in maintaining the num-ber of supplements you are taking comparatively low, you can correct your nutritional regimen so. For example, if you consume lots of fatty, cold-water fish, then you might not have to supplement using omega-3 fatty acids. Consider your daily diet and nutritional supplement in a proper method to ensure you're giving your body exactly what it requires.

Here is one important note to remember while you're considering nutritional supplements: Your daily recommended allowances for vitamins, minerals, nutritional supplements, and other chemicals that you see on food labels do not indicate a great deal. These tips show you the minimum quantities necessary for the body to keep working properly. However, they do not let you know exactly what amounts you will need for the body to really go beyond and above that foundation level.

## Multiminerals

In general, you will need to provide your system using 16 distinct nutritional supplements if you would like it to perform at an optimum level.

Multimineral nutritional supplements are simple to discover, and in several instances, you are able to discover multivitamin/multi-mineral combination nutritional supplements. These options can be challenging, and you have to be certain if you decide to go that path, you purchase an option that comprises all 14 vitamins along with all 16 nutritional supplements. (That is rather a good deal!)

If you are picking a multi-mineral supplement, then go with one which features chelated minerals. I will spare you all of the full details of this procedure, which produces chelated minerals. But remember that unless you are getting chelated minerals, then you are likely paying for nutritional supplements that wind up on your bathroom rather than on your own body's major systems.

Do not choose a multi-mineral supplement that arrives out of a clay resource. These goods aren't chelated, plus they feature tin, silver, and nickel. Sometimes they even record lead as a component!

## Omega-3 Fatty Acids

You have probably read or heard about omega-3 fatty acids in the news lately. The significance of this essential fatty acid was getting a great deal of press, also for great reason. It is one of these substances your body needs to endure and flourish. Despite all of the wonderfully intricate chemical processes that your own body can perform, it cannot fabricate omega-3 fatty acids.

The best dietary source of omega-3s is beef. Fish is another great resource. You ought to consume fish as part of a proper diet; however, unless you are eating wild Alaskan salmon, or even among those other few kinds of fish that do not commonly contain elevated levels of mercury, it is likely that you're becoming an extremely salty dose of toxins with your own omega-3 fatty acids.

To stay clear of germs but nevertheless get your omega-3 supplement, use liquid fish oil or even some capsule or soft gel. Take 1 g twice per day to get exactly what you want.

## Resveratrol

Resveratrol is a highly effective antioxidant, and I recommend that everybody get a dose of this every day. Resveratrol has generated a higher profile as a Harvard Medical School case study. A couple of years back, it was revealed that a fairly dramatic gain in mice's health and lifespan after they have been given resveratrol. If you read about this particular antioxidant, you will likely see that it is in red wine, which is reality. However, if you wished to receive an important dose of resveratrol from red wine, you'd need to glug a couple of hundred bottles of the material daily, which will kill you before you have to enjoy the advantages of resveratrol.

The fantastic thing is you can purchase resveratrol supplements in many health food shops and in any vitamin store, either in person or on the internet. You will find it labeled either as resveratrol or red wine extract. I suggest getting 30 mg every day that ought to be somewhat simple, given the width of nutritional supplement options available in the industry.

## Vitamin C

If you choose a fantastic multivitamin, then you are likely to get a fantastic amount of vitamin C every day. But do not believe for a moment you are getting all your body should truly have the ability to work on a top degree.

I suggest carrying a 1,000-milligram vitamin C supplement two times every day. I know that seems like a great deal, but if you've read about it, you understand why I believe very strongly that vitamin C is a massive blessing for your great health. Though it's within plenty of vegetables and fruits, it may continue to be hard to get enough of the things on your diet plan. Hundreds (maybe thousands) of vitamin C supplement options are available, so do some research and speak with your naturopathic physician to discover which ones are ideal for you.

If you are fighting a disease, take 8,000 mg of vitamin C daily rather than the normal 2,000 mg.

## Vitamin B Complex

The term vitamin B complex describes all the vitamins B: B1, B2, B3, B5, B6, B7, B9, and B12. A number of the vitamins B also have several other widely used titles—riboflavin and niacin are just two great examples.

The assortment of important features the vitamin B complex performs on the human body is shocking, and I would not even try to cover all the details. Just know that in the event you would like to be healthy and live a long, comfy lifestyle, you had better concentrate on getting lots of vitamins B.

It's a fantastic idea to have a vitamin B complex supplement as well as a multivitamin daily. You'll be able to discover such a supplement that can provide you exactly what you need in just one dose every day.

## Sulforaphane

Not everybody has heard of sulforaphane, and that is too bad. It has been making headlines on a fairly regular basis recently, and everybody ought to be carrying it as a nutritional supplement regularly.

Recent studies have suggested that sulforaphane will help thwart some sorts of cancer and may slow tumor growth. Additional studies reveal that sulforaphane lessens the quantity of H. pylori bacteria from the gut, which is what triggers stomach lining inflammation and nausea. If those are not good reasons to choose sulforaphane every day, I do not understand what exactly they are.

You're able to get sulforaphane in supplement form in 2 manners: carrot seed infusion or plain sulforaphane. If you go for the latter, then take 500 mg daily. In case the prior is the favorite sulforaphane nutritional supplement, attempt to receive 30 mg daily.

## Vitamin E

Along with vitamin C and vitamin B complex, vitamin E is something that will almost surely be included in your multivitamin routine but likely not in large enough quantities. You'll be able to see continuing health benefits of supplementing with vitamin E around 800 mg every day and therefore don't be reluctant to take that much.

What are a few of the health advantages of taking extra vitamin E? To begin with, vitamin E has strong antioxidant effects. But vitamin E does a number of other fantastic things for the body, too, from boosting your immune system to maintaining blood vessels at tiptop form.

Do yourself a massive favor and do not scrimp on the vitamin E.

### Alpha-Lipoic Acid (ALA)

You will frequently see the lipoic acid known as ALA. It is a top-notch antioxidant that helps your body fight infection and retains your cells working at a higher level.

Choose an ALA nutritional supplement and locate a capsule type that produces about 800 mg every day. That amount was demonstrated to provide many health benefits with no overpowering or side-effects within the human body. It's possible to locate ALA supplements in any fantastic health food shop and in the regional vitamin retailer.

## DR. SEBI HERBAL TEAS

### Herbal Teas

Burdock Tea – Select some fresh chunks of burdock root. They need to be somewhat firm and not too soft. The color can range from a light color like parchment paper to a dark brown that looks like tree bark. Only buy the root you can use immediately for tea, because they do not keep very well. Any leftover root should be put into a soup. If you chose a younger root, you could simply rinse it well, but an older root will need the outer skin scraped off. If you can't source fresh root, you can use one tablespoon of dried root that has been aged for at least one year. If you are using fresh root, then you will need two tablespoons of the root coarsely chopped. Boil the root with three cups of filtered water, and then let it simmer for thirty minutes. Move the pot from the heat and let the tea steep for another thirty minutes. Drink the tea to detox your body

Chamomile Tea – This is an herbal infusion that is made from the dried flowers of the chamomile plant steeped in water. Only Roman Chamomile and German Chamomile are used to make tea. This tea is naturally devoid of caffeine and is often used as a sleep aid. Gather four tablespoons of fresh chamomile flowers, one small sprig of fresh mint, and eight ounces (one cup) of boiling water. Chamomile flowers should ideally be used the same day they are harvested to get the best flavor and medicinal benefits. You will want a tea ball, tea infuser, or a cheesecloth pouch to put the chamomile flowers and mint sprig in. Boil the water and then add in the flowers and mint. Allow the tea at least five minutes to steep. If needed, you can put the mint sprig and the chamomile flowers directly into the water while you boil and steep the tea, and then strain the tea well before drinking. Drink this tea to help you sleep.

Elderberry Tea – This is a delicious tea with the power to boost your immune system. Gather two cups of filtered water, one teaspoon of honey, one-half teaspoon of turmeric powder, one-half teaspoon of cinnamon, and two tablespoons of dried elderberries. Place the elderberries into a small saucepan with the filtered water and blend in the cinnamon and turmeric. Bring this to boiling and then let it simmer for fifteen minutes. The simmering will help to bring out the healing properties of the elderberries. Strain the tea water into a cup and blend in the honey as you desire. If you prefer this tea to be served cold, simply refrigerate it after straining or pour it over ice cubes. Drink elderberry tea when you feel a cold or flu coming on.

Fennel Tea – This is a good tea to drink when you have a digestive upset. Gather two teaspoons of fennel seeds, one cup of water, one teaspoon of dried lemon verbena, and one teaspoon of ginger that has been freshly grated. Crush the fennel seeds to release their healing compounds. Peel the chunk of ginger before you grate it. Add all of the ingredients into the water in a small saucepan and boil, and then let it simmer for ten minutes. Strain the tea and drink it immediately. Drink this tea whenever you need to soothe an upset stomach.

Ginger Tea – This is another tea to boost your immunity. It will also warm you in cold weather without giving you caffeine jitters. Rinse off the ginger root to remove any visible dirt. You don't need to peel the root unless you want to. Slice the ginger root, using about an inch of root for eight ounces of water. Put the water and the ginger root in a saucepan and boil, and then simmer for ten minutes. Strain the hot tea and drop in a slice of lemon and a teaspoon of honey for flavor. Drink ginger tea any time your stomach or digestive system needs a little extra help.

Raspberry Tea – This tea is best served cold to get the best flavor. Use a large pot to boil four quarts of water with one and one-half cups of sugar. Take the pot from the heat and keep stirring until all of the sugar is dissolved. Put in twelve ounces of raspberries, ten regular tea bags, and one-fourth cup of lemon juice. Cover the pot and let all of this steep for ten minutes. Then strain the tea well and serve it over ice or refrigerate the tea until it is cold. Drink this tea to stay well hydrated.

Tila (Linden) Tea – This is one of the simplest of the herbal tea recipes. Add one tablespoon of dried linden flowers in a tea ball or mesh basket to three cups (twenty-four ounces) of boiling water. If you need to put the linden flowers directly in the water, just strain it well before drinking it. Cover the container and let the flowers steep for at least fifteen minutes. You can add honey to sweeten the tea if you desire, and feel free to drink this tea freely to soothe frazzled nerves.

# DR. SEBI'S CURE FOR HERPES

## WHAT IS HERPES SIMPLEX VIRUS?

A significant outbreak is usually more severe than the subsequent ones. When the initial attack is over, it becomes inactive and does not cause symptoms again. This period is known as the dormant infection; at any point after this, the herpes virus can pop up again. It then becomes reactive and once again causes sores.

The frequency, severity, and duration of outbreaks can significantly be reduced with herbal treatments and mixtures.

People with HSV-2 virus may experience any of the following:

- Significant burning and itching while urinating
- Chills, fever, headaches, flu-like symptoms, and body aches
- Swollen lymph nodes in the groin area
- Pain or discomfort around the legs, genitals, or buttocks
- Constipation, or difficulty while urinating

The best way to verify—if you think you've been exposed to the herpes virus is to go for a test because you may experience no symptoms.

Most people may not have figured out the exact cause of their breakup. Most warning signs include:

- Tingling
- Numbness
- Tenderness

Itching around the area where the sores will appear

There can also be pains near the back of the legs, lower back, and buttocks. There often start a few hours to days before the actual sores appear on the patient's skin.

Sores can re-appear near the genital or in places where it has appeared before. There has been much advancement to help individuals who suffer from genital herpes. This advancement comes in the form of herbal treatments and supplements. Many compounds have been found in nature that reduce HSV-2 outbreaks, duration, and frequency. Most of these treatments aren't affiliated with the big pharmaceutical companies; these natural remedies are typically affordable and can be accessed from anywhere around the globe.

### Herpes Zoster

Herpes zoster is the clinical manifestation of the Varicella Zoster virus's reactivation, the primary infection of chickenpox, an exanthemata disease affecting mainly children. It is characterized by maculae, bumps and blisters, and crusts. The viral DNA finds shelter in the posterior sensory ganglia or the cranial pars. Different factors comprising stress, immune depression, lymphomas, or immunosuppressive drugs may trigger the activation of this genetic material and progress towards the epidermis. This triggering effect can take place at any time. However, it prevails in people who are older or have a depressed immune system. It is not season-related.

## Varicella-Zoster Virus

The VZV belongs to the Herpes virus family and comprises a double-chain DNA genome with a lipoprotein layer that helps the virus adhere and get into.

It gains access through the airway and replicates in the ganglia of the rachidian nerves, resulting in the first viridian.

## Chickenpox or first infection

The virus gains access through the respiratory epithelium and replicates in the lymph nodes, spreading through the blood and resulting in chickenpox. Symptoms do not take more than 15 days. The virus remains inside the posterior lymph nodes.

How Can I Contract the Disease?

From saliva, HSV-1 or oral herpes is transmitted.

Via interaction with genital secretions, herpes blisters, & mucosal surfaces, HSV-2 or genital herpes is spread. Both viruses can also be released from skin or mucosa that do not tend to have signs or to be contaminated.

The individual must refrain from oral, anal, or vaginal sex with someone affected with HSV-2 to avoid contractions with genital herpes. To do this, you should abstain from sex entirely or have sex in a legally monogamous partnership in which neither spouse exhibits genital herpes.

The use of contraceptives might even minimize the risk of genital herpes, but lesions could be present in places that are not covered by condoms, and no lesions need to be visible for the disease to spread. Some strategies to avoid or minimize the transmission of the infection can involve taking medicine each day to prevent an epidemic, or after an epidemic, avoiding participating in anal, oral, or vaginal intercourse uses?

What are the Causes of Herpes?

There are some primary causes of herpes, which I am going to talk about below:

## Oral sex

Oral sex is good, and I do not deny it, but it is wise for us to know who and how healthy our partner's mouth is. If the mouth of the person giving you a leader has cold sores around his/her mouth, there is a tendency that you might get infected with herpes.

## Unprotected sex

Having unprotected sex with someone suffering from herpes transmits the virus.

*Transmitted through birth*

Another craziest thing about this virus is that it can be transmitted from the mother to her newborn baby through birth delivery if the mother's genital herpes have sores while giving birth.

Please note that the sharing of towels, chairs, kitchen utensils, or toilet seats with someone with herpes cannot get you infected because the viruses need a moist environment to be transmitted. That is why it can be transmitted through the eyes, anus, vagina, mouth, and wounds.

*What are the Common Symptoms of Herpes?*

Many people are carrying this virus without showing any symptoms, but some people have their signs, and such people can develop them within 2–12 days after they are exposed to the virus.

However, whenever someone is exposed to the virus for the first time, the virus's recurrences tend to happen more frequently, but the remission periods get longer as time goes on. Each occurrence of the virus tends to become less severe.

## HERPES AND RELATIONSHIPS

*Being Able to Understand A Person with Herpes*

Are you unable to understand what type of person we are talking with because herpes is a virus that can cause discomfort in the person? We will give you some tips that you can use so that this disease won't obstruct your perspective.

Herpes is a virus that creates discomfort in the person. It can be transmitted from one person to another through skin-to-skin contact. The virus then reproduces in the cells nearest to where it entered and soon moves to other parts of the body. The first outbreak of herpes may cause fever, headache, muscle aches, and a painful sore throat. Herpes is not just an uncomfortable health condition. Still, it also makes people less welcoming by making them unwilling to speak about their state with others for fear of rejection or embarrassment.

But does being herpes mean you need to be judged? Not at all. Once exposed to the virus, the body's immune system usually takes care of it, limiting its impact and severity. If a person's first episode of genital herpes is mild, he or she might never notice it was occurring. Those who do get symptoms usually appear within two weeks after contact with the virus and last up to 3 weeks. These blisters break open and leave sores that may take 2 to 4 weeks to heal completely.

These treatments work best when applied at the first sign of tingling or itching. Using these creams, however, will not prevent the spread of herpes to others.

Once someone has been infected with herpes, they may have no more outbreaks or just infrequent ones. Medications can be taken to help control outbreaks. There are two types of drugs used to treat herpes, acyclovir, and valacyclovir. These drugs help prevent attacks or shorten the time they last, but they do not cure herpes infections.

The stigma surrounding herpes is more similar to past stigmas against homosexuality than it is to celiac disease or AIDS; those conditions are harmful in demonstrably correct ways while being branded as "undesirable" by an entire culture only makes someone feel bad about themselves and discourages them from being who they are.

Having herpes means you have a virus that's capable of causing symptoms. This virus can be very mild or extremely severe, depending on the route of entry.

Herpes is a common occurrence that affects millions of people, and many people are not even aware that they have it. According to Zeigler & Anderson, approximately 20 million people in the United States are currently infected with herpes. That is around 1 out of 8 Americans. The Centers for Disease Control and Prevention estimate that 45 million Americans have herpes simplex virus (HSV).

Herpes causes pain in the mouth/face and genitals and causes blisters or sores on your skin. However, herpes is more of a nuisance than an illness. There is no cure for herpes yet, but you can take drugs to ease the symptoms and prevent outbreaks.

Herpes simplex is a viral infection that causes painful blisters or sores on the mouth or genitals. It was once thought to be hereditary only, but recent research suggests that everyone carries the virus in their body, but it will not cause symptoms in most people. Herpes affects at least 50 million Americans, with one out of every six people between 14 and 49 years old infected with some form of genital herpes. Most people who carry the HSV-1 virus between outbreaks have few if any symptoms.

Although a friend could ask us if we have ever had herpes, to be honest, we feel that it is better not to know. Once you know about the disease, you cannot read about someone with a similar illness and not compare yourself. People often think that someone who has been diagnosed with herpes must be the wrong person or an addict.

When we get tested for an STD, we will be told what type of disease it is. However, many people in the world cannot tell their diagnosis to others because of their shame and embarrassment. It is our responsibility to share this information with everyone who may be troubled by this disease. We will give you tips that may help you and offer some advice from other people who have been living with herpes for years. Please read through some of these tips and see if you can find some that will help you deal with your illness better.

The doctor said that the disease was herpes. However, he didn't give me any information and told me to ask my friends. I don't know anyone diagnosed with an STD, so I wondered how to get some help. No one wants to talk about this subject because they are afraid that others will think they are bad people.

There is a "life after herpes," but no one would believe you if you say this. However, if we do not act as nothing happened and move on with our lives, it is possible to have herpes without letting it stop us from doing what we need to do every day. Indeed, some people can't even go to work because they are infected with this virus. Some people do not have a job since having herpes may affect the things that they do.

In the US, it is said that there are over 3 million people who are diagnosed with herpes and about 11,000 new cases diagnosed every year. It is also said that about 500,000 Americans have herpes, but they don't know it since they haven't been tested, and there's no cure for them yet.

A young man who was an amicable and intelligent person had this disease. It was a shame that he couldn't tell others about his herpes diagnosis because he felt like they would be disgusted when they heard it. The only thing this man knew to do was to find another person who also had herpes. This way, he wouldn't feel lonely and embarrassed without anyone to talk with him.

Since herpes is not curable, someone might say that it is better not to have it in the first place. However, you should not be ashamed of your disease or hide the fact that you have gotten an STD since most of them can still live happily even if they are infected with an STD.

Herpes is a common STD that can affect people of all ages. For some people, their body is strongly influenced by these symptoms, and they will see them even after they have been cured. Others might be fortunate in this aspect and reduce the amount of physical discomfort associated with the disease. There is no cure for herpes since it requires a lifetime medication to prevent germs from forming, which would spread it again in the future.

What are some essential things that we should do when we have been diagnosed with herpes?

Your friends might be surprised if you tell them that you have herpes but don't make any attempts to hide it from them. Many people in the world are afraid of getting into an accident because they have severe disease, but they will feel great if they can convince themselves that this will not happen to them for sure.

Herpes can be treated with ointments and medications, so if you stay diligent and monitor its progress, then you should be able to manage it easily. Although there is no cure for herpes yet, doctors can help us keep our condition by taking care of it every day.

In one of my college classes, I met a boy who was diagnosed with herpes. It was the first time that I had heard of the disease, and it made quite an impression on me. They would be tested for this disease shortly, and then he would start getting treatment for it. At first, it was extraordinary that he didn't tell anyone about his diagnosis because usually, people are more comfortable talking about it rather than keeping quiet about something like this.

Most people have no idea what to do when they find out that they have herpes. They often do not tell anyone about their diagnosis because they are afraid of getting a negative response from those around them.

People often get disturbed when faced with the problem of herpes since it is a severe disease that can affect their daily lives in many ways. Although there is no cure for herpes yet, we can still control it by taking medications meant for this purpose. It is essential to avoid having unprotected sex since it can help the virus to spread.

Herpes can cause a lot of physical discomforts and mental distress. It is important not to let this disease take control over your life, so you need to know how to treat it and get relief from the symptoms that are bothering you. I'm going to share some valuable tips on how to get rid of herpes and get back your life again for ordinary people like us. If you are not well-informed about this disease, it will be harder for you to diagnose it correctly, and no one will be able to help you treat it appropriately.

Some doctors and clinics can help you get rid of herpes, but you should know that some of them charge quite a high amount of money. It is essential to find a doctor or clinic that will help you treat your disease without charging for the services they provide.

Many people don't know how to treat it properly, becoming more agitated every day. There are many different symptoms associated with this disease, so if your discomfort increases over time.

## Herpes Stigma: The Fear of People

There is no reason to be embarrassed or ashamed of having Herpes. It's not a death sentence, it's not contagious, and it doesn't make you dirty. There are many other myths about the disease that people believe, and that is just plain false. Once you know what herpes is all about, you'll feel much more confident in your decision-making and in how to handle social situations with this condition.

That's where the downfall begins! No matter how many times a day you pray to God for help, how much money you spend on ineffective treatments, or how many doctors visit, it won't get rid of it! You're missing the two most important factors in dealing with a disease like this - education and a positive mental attitude.

Herpes stigma is a complex topic to talk about, but we must do it.

Luckily, there's a lot of information out there about herpes and how to fight the stigma so that one day we can start seeing genital herpes as just another benign condition in life. If you have genital herpes or have ever come into contact with someone who does, no matter what gender they are or anything else — then you'll be glad you read this!

Don't be scared — because being educated is your best weapon against herpes stigma.

## Impact Of Herpes Stigma

Herpes stigma is a term for the negative attitudes or beliefs that one person may hold about those with herpes. Stigma can affect an individual's thoughts, feelings, and behaviors in many ways, such as limiting their social interactions or causing them to experience intense feelings of shame and isolation.

The stigma of herpes has been a significant part of the problem for many people and is often why many people who have it do not get tested. There are so many misconceptions about herpes out there that it might be challenging to know where to start.

But first things first: how every day is herpes? Up to one in four adults in the US has genital HSV-2, and up to 90% of those infected don't know they have it. Of course, HSV-1 causes cold sores, but most people infected with that strain don't even realize it.

Herpes is a widespread virus, and yet there's so much misinformation out there. One of the main reasons for this stigma is that people don't understand its spread and how it can be prevented. For example, many people think herpes can only be spread during an outbreak. About 90% of new infections occur when someone is not experiencing symptoms or signs. Even if your partner has never had a cold sore or another outbreak, you could still transmit the virus to them by skin-to-skin contact when you have no symptoms or signs that you're shedding the virus (such as when you're on your period).

The virus is probably most easily transmitted when there are visible sores, but people can spread the virus without even knowing it. One of the more important things to remember is that a person with herpes may not be aware that they have it. They may have contracted it from someone else and be unaware that they are now a carrier. Most people get herpes due to having sex with someone infected, but neither partner has symptoms! If you had a partner who never disclosed their infection to you, would you want to know? Or would you prefer to remain unknowing?

For many, herpes comes as quite a shock and can leave them feeling insecure about their bodies and self-worth. This can lead to decreased self-esteem and shame, and it can also act as a barrier to getting tested. People are often reluctant to disclose their condition to their doctors, especially if they have had negative experiences in the past. Besides, herpes is listed as one of those infections that people will lie about if you ask them about it.

At any point during an outbreak or after your symptoms have disappeared, you may still be contagious and spreading the virus even though your sores haven't healed yet. If you are diagnosed with herpes, it's essential to know that you don't have to identify yourself as a person with herpes or share this information with other people. No one has to know you have herpes, and no one will know---unless you tell them.

Besides, there are now over a dozen new medications on the market that can reduce or eliminate outbreaks. When taken daily, these medications make it much easier for those who have the virus to manage their condition alone. Some people may not experience any outbreaks at all!

You can also do things to reduce the risk of spreading herpes to your partner, such as taking suppressive medications daily. Condoms can also help prevent transmission as long as they're worn correctly. Be sure to check with your doctor or pharmacist about what medications are right for you and learn how to make condoms fit for maximum protection.

The stigma associated with herpes can significantly impact those who are diagnosed, but that doesn't mean people have to suffer alone.

The stigma of herpes has been a significant part of the problem for many people and is often why many people who have it do not get tested. There are so many misconceptions about herpes out there that it might be challenging to know where to start. But first things first: how every day is herpes? Up to one in four adults in the US has genital HSV-2, and up to 90% of those infected don't know they have it. Of course, HSV-1 causes cold sores, but most people infected with that strain don't even realize it. The virus is probably most easily transmitted when there are visible sores, but people can spread the virus without even knowing it. One of the more important things to remember is that a person with herpes may not be aware that they have it. They may have contracted it from someone else and be unaware that they are now a carrier. Most people get herpes due to having sex with someone infected, but neither partner has symptoms! If you had a partner who never disclosed their infection to you, would you want to know? Or would you prefer to remain unknowing? At any point during an outbreak or after your symptoms have disappeared, you may still be contagious and spreading the virus even though your sores haven't healed yet. If you are diagnosed with herpes, it's essential to know that you don't have to identify yourself as a person with herpes or share this information with other people. No one has to know you have herpes, and no one will know---unless you tell them. Besides, there are now over a dozen new medications on the market that can reduce or eliminate outbreaks. When taken daily, these medications make it much easier for those who have the virus to manage their condition alone. Some people may not experience any outbreaks at all! You can also do things to reduce the risk of spreading herpes to your partner, such as taking suppressive medications daily. Condoms can also help prevent transmission as long as they're worn correctly. Be sure to check with your doctor or pharmacist about what medications are right for you and learn how to make condoms fit for maximum protection. The stigma associated with herpes can significantly impact those who are diagnosed, but that doesn't mean people have to suffer alone.

The impact of herpes stigma on those living with genital herpes can be significant. It may lead to difficulties in accessing health care services and medical information because of fear of discrimination; it is a common reason for opting out from preventative counseling during STI screens; it may also lead to increased rates of unprotected sex among those who are not fully aware that they are infected with HSV-1 or HSV-2.

Many people who have herpes believe that their condition is incredibly shameful and often suffer in silence, but want to let people know about their own experiences living with the virus. Herpes stigma is also present in society, where individuals may feel shame for having contracted HSV-1 or HSV-2. Both types of HSV can be spread through skin-to-skin contact, which occurs during outbreaks or simply due to having the virus because it remains in a person's body even when they are not experiencing an attack.

Stigma conveys a sense of disgrace and has been used to marginalize groups of people. Historically, it has been used to justify the oppression of certain groups and individuals. In the case of those with herpes, it is often associated with sexual promiscuity and infidelity.

Stigma may also lead to fear of rejection by others, including sexual partners or future employers; it can hurt the quality of life and self-esteem; it may cause difficulty in securing employment or housing, and in some cases can lead to psychological illness such as depression. Stigma may also cause those who are infected to believe that they must keep their infection secret from family members, friends, or other loved ones -- potentially causing further isolation. Additionally, people may not disclose because they believe that others will react negatively towards them.

## What is Herpes Stigma?

Herpes stigma is negative attitudes and beliefs about people with herpes, which causes them to be discriminated against. This wrong notion makes people treat them like they are socially unacceptable or second-class citizens.

Some of the challenges herpes patients get to endure include:

Discrimination from healthcare professionals cause of their status

## Social isolation or distancing

People are refusing to make contact with the cause of their status.

This sort of treatment has made people diagnosed with herpes recoil into their shells or even consider the diagnosis as a sexual death sentence and often relegate themselves to a life of celibacy afterward. Sometimes, even the health care provider doesn't help matters because of how they cast these looks that screams, 'You should have known better.' And as a result of this stigma, most end up not talking about it and suffer psychologically and emotionally in silence.

In truth, most of the stigma that comes from herpes, as with other sexually transmitted diseases, comes from fear and misinformation. Also, the general lack of sex education among the populace hasn't made matters easy. Data collected by CDC shows that over 776,000 in the US are diagnosed with herpes annually, and over 12% of its populace aged 14 to 49 have the infection. Yet you wonder why, even with this high number why the stigma still stands.

Basic sex education classes would always advise that abstinence is the best policy; much more comprehensive studies would always ask that periodic tests be done among sexually active people. The whole system still fails to give any advice on what to do in the event a person tests positive and, as a result, leaves most clueless and in fear of what others might think of them.

## Living with Herpes Stigma

The stigma surrounding herpes can be debilitating. Even if you don't have herpes, you may feel the need to watch what you say around people who do. We're here to show you that living with herpes doesn't have to be a source of shame or embarrassment. It can even provide an important lesson about love and relationships. Why? Because as ridiculous and outdated as some of the stigmas is, it's impossible to talk about living with herpes without talking about sex.

Just like any other STD, there are ways that people live successful lives while managing a chronic condition such as herpes - no matter how much society wants us to believe otherwise.

As a teenager, I grew up in a small town. While my friends explored their sexuality by experimenting with contraceptive methods and various forms of birth control, I was too embarrassed to bother. When the time came to start dating, I was resistant to physical relationships because of the stigma surrounding herpes. Unfortunately, it took an infection to kindle a spark of awareness when nothing would have changed for me otherwise. I'm living proof that living with herpes doesn't have to be complicated or embarrassing.

Our lives are full of complicated decisions and decisions that have life-altering consequences. I made mine so long ago when I decided to keep my herpes to myself.

I want to make it clear: choosing to stay with someone with whom you have herpes does not mean that you will automatically transmit herpes or even develop symptoms. Having an STD does not equal becoming infected or developing symptoms for everyone who has them.

Let me break it down for you:

For many people who have herpes but don't know they do, the virus can lie dormant without causing an outbreak. For others, the virus is active but asymptomatic. Symptoms may be obvious, or they may be so subtle that you don't notice them at all. The point is that having herpes in your system doesn't mean that you will have symptoms that are visible to someone else or even that you'll transmit the virus to a partner who doesn't have it already.

It's impossible to know for sure what will happen if you have unprotected sex with someone who has herpes. I know this isn't what anyone wants to hear. It certainly wasn't what I wanted to hear when I was younger.

Let me be honest: we weren't always practicing safe sex. It took a few partners before I learned the facts about herpes and how it can be transmitted. The first time my partner told me that he had herpes, it came out of nowhere and nearly destroyed our relationship. I'm ashamed to say that I couldn't tell you that there was even such a thing as non-genital herpes (cold sores) before him.

I was sheltered from all forms of sexual education and remained ignorant about herpes until my high school years. This lack of knowledge about herpes when it came to my relationships led me to make some questionable decisions regarding dating and having sex.

While feeling completely ashamed, I would often justify my actions by saying that it wasn't that big of a deal because "everyone knows" that herpes is an STD. This embarrassment and fear made me keep information about myself and my health so closely guarded.

I found out about the symptoms of herpes and why they aren't contagious but remained utterly unaware of how to take care of myself if I ever became infected. There were no sex ed classes in high school, and no one from my friends' families ever talked about STDs or told us what to do if we were ever in an intimate relationship with someone who has them.

While it's easy for me to laugh at myself now, these are the very kinds of decisions that give others pause when it comes to having sex with someone who may have herpes.

They weren't sexually active herself at the time and knew very little about it. While she was dating him, he got an outbreak and didn't tell her about it to fear how she'd react. When word got out (in a small town, information spreads fast), everyone began to talk about him like a leper that no one wanted to be caught dead with. And the worst part of all? He still didn't know that his outbreaks were contagious during an attack.

He had an understandable reaction of shame and denial. He decided that was in his best interest: he broke up with my friend and lied to her about why. She, in turn, was heartbroken and ended up losing both him and their friendship.

Why? Because like me back then, she couldn't keep it together when someone she cared about had herpes. She didn't understand how a person could be so cruel to someone who had done nothing wrong, someone, with whom they were intimate. Years later, I asked her if she would ever let anyone know if she found out that she had herpes and learned about the symptoms of herpes for the first time. She said she would never tell anyone.

When confronted with this information, I'm sure some will say, "Well, you just shouldn't have been having sex with him in the first place." And I can't deny that. But what if that were the only available option? If the only way you could protect yourself from herpes was to avoid sex? What then?

Again, I realize this is a thought that many people won't want to hear. But again, let me be honest: it's difficult not to judge someone who is having unprotected sex with someone who doesn't know how herpes is transmitted -- especially when they're in a relationship.

Herpes is a sexually transmitted infection with a stigma that is so huge, and it could practically swallow the sunBut if you don't want to transmit herpes to your partner (or vice versa), then you'll need communication and protection with each other.

We're not saying that herpes is no big deal; it's an important one. But forget all the negativity surrounding herpes. Show your partner that herpes is no big deal.

Just think of "herpes" as a tiny little dot on your hand. It doesn't hurt you, and you can't see it unless your hands are touching each other or inanimate objects. It can also occur if someone touches an infected area without clean hands first (or even without realizing they have an infection).

Let me explain. The first, HSV-1, is the more common and usually the more severe. This form often causes an outbreak of herpes around the mouth area but can also cause explosions around the waist and legs. Sexually transmitted herpes can affect as many as one in six Americans, and it's spreading faster than ever before. One small study done in 2004 show that one in three women has herpes caused by HSV-1 during pregnancy, and one in five pregnant women have genital herpes. Of course, this means that this rate likely increases with every passing year.

When you think about it, this doesn't sound too alarming. After all, if one in three women has herpes because of HSV-1, two in three women don't have it. The problem is that HSV-1 is relatively easy to spread, especially when you're having symptoms of herpes. Why? Because most people don't even know they have it.

Most of the time with HSV-1, you won't ever know you have contracted the disease because the symptoms are mild. It usually doesn't show up for months or years after transmission.

The herpes virus is not fatal, but people who are affected often experience moderate to severe discomfort and pain. Some people experienced death due to the virus, but it only happens when they contact children (who have weaker immune systems) during the outbreak phase.

It's important to know that there has not been a case of transmission based on handshakes or hugs because this usually does not involve any direct contact of fluids from one person to another.

There are a stigma and lack of knowledge surrounding herpes, making it difficult for people to find the information they need to live healthy lives. With so many infected across the world, one in five people, it's essential that we provide easy access to this much-needed information. This article aims to bring awareness and understanding about this widespread infection.

Talk about uncomfortable! But if you know someone who might be infected with an STI, or if you're someone who may have been living with an undiagnosed STI, then please read on!

The prevalence of sexually transmitted infections is astounding. All well know this staggering statistic.

But what isn't as widely talked about is the stigma and social taboo associated with STIs. Many people still think of STIs as a congenital disability or life-long disability, when in fact, they're treatable and curable. Others refuse to get tested because they expect to be "cured." They think that the testing will be unneeded after a few months, and they go without knowing their status — and possibly infect others.

The good news is that most adults are immune to the virus. If you have not been exposed to it, you will not contract it. That's why you have to get tested if anyone suggests that you may have been. You may end up having false results and start taking medications when you don't need to.

## DR. SEBI'S METHOD FOR TREATING HERPES

Humans have been acquainted with various types of medicines, among which we have homeopathy, allopathy, natural medication, and a few different treatments. Homeopathy is a treatment that regards an individual all in all. After a case-investigation and individual assessment, homeopathic remedies are chosen, which incorporates a clinical history check, mental and physical constitution, and so on. This implies homeopathic treatment centers around the patient as an individual, just as his unstable condition.

Allopathy, then again, is the study of rewarding maladies with variable cures, not the same as the impact of the ailment itself. This type of treatment has been the standard in past decades. Individuals wholeheartedly acknowledged this treatment without posing inquiries concerning its source, dependability, and impacts. This type of treatment keeps on flourishing because of the large number of dollars that pharmaceutical organizations spend on commercials yearly. Both of these frameworks have been attempted. However, they have not been able to fix herpes infection forever on the human body. This makes them off-limits territory for herpes patients. To the extent rewarding herpes is your primary need, all the antiviral medications you have been spending on so far will do little to nothing to help free your collection of herpes. The impacts given by these medications can be effortlessly acquired by some different methods, an elective that will free you of the side effects and the reactions.

Regular medication has given us no other option than to go to traditional techniques. The equivalent conventional daily practice for a herpes fix watched decades back is despite everything being followed today to fix herpes. The far-reaching of herpes throughout the years has made discovering its hole a worldwide concern. As the infection keeps on plaguing millions worldwide, another settlement has been reached, that is, to go to the traditional remedy for herpes over conventional medication.

Realities About Dr. Sebi's Method to Cure Herpes

In contrast to customary specialists, Dr. Sebi didn't see maladies and sicknesses due to germs intrusion, bacterial contamination, or an infection. To him, it is all a matter of where and when the mucous film has been undermined. Contingent upon the sight, the illnesses can be effortlessly arranged. Dr. Sebi is famous for restoring the most feared diseases like notorious malignancy, herpes infection, hypertension, diabetes, and numerous ailments.

Every other disorder that has been known to be hopeless by specialists everywhere throughout the world can be relieved by Dr. Sebi's herpes fix. You're eating routine will be as per what your invulnerable framework cherishes and what the infection despises. The food will, for the most part, contain each supplement your body needs to remain dynamic.

Eat a more incredible amount of Dr. Sebi's suggested products of the soil, sodas, sweet, and greasy nourishments. Eat less of the accompanying or thoroughly avoid them during flare-ups:

- Almonds
- Cashews
- Corn
- Meat
- Nuts (except for the ones suggested by dr. Sebi)
- Barley
- Cereals
- Chicken
- Oats and peanuts

The mentioned contain l-arginine, an amino corrosive that stifles l-lysine, the amino corrosive that is answerable for hindering the development pace of the infection. However much as could be expected, Attempt to keep away from these during your disease stage and after. There is a particular basic eating routine that Dr. Sebi exclusively roused. It is pointed towards giving the body alkalizing nourishments that decline bodily fluid with Dr. Sebi's herpes fix. The rationale behind this fix is the formation of a poisonous situation to the herpes infection, one in which it thinks that it's hard to develop. For this to occur, you have to eat nourishments that are toxic to the disease. This motivating force involves taking spices and Dr. Sebi's homegrown oil, a superior option compared to taking the harmful antivirals, which are just fit for harming the body. Dr. Sebi's herpes fix is explicitly intended to assault the cell structure of the herpes simplex infection, in this way giving you a herpes-free life.

The indications for herpes disease are now and then "trickish" and unnoticeable, making herpes patients not realize they have to see a specialist; for other people, the manifestations are extreme. They generally show inside possibly 14 days of interacting with the infection. Once in a while, the side effects would disappear in a couple of days, while on different occasions, the manifestations continue for up to a month. Herpes victims can identify with this experience.

## Curing Herpes Via Dr. Sebi's Food Plan

Dr. Sebi frequently referred to that to heal the frame. Dr. Sebi contends that "diseases" cannot live in an alkaline frame, and so it's far vital to cleanse and alkalize the body to carry it to a more fit state.

Step 1 Smooth up the Machine

Detoxifying the gadget is pivotal to freeing the edge of ailments. To start with, we begin with the guide of purging out the colon (entrails).

## Colon cleanse

Use chelation 2 for this. You can make your own if you can't buy it. There also are other techniques for cleaning the colon and cleansing out the bowel. Any appropriate colon cleanses recipe needs to assist.

## Apple Onion Colon Cleanse Recipe

Preparation time: 10 Minutes

Cooking time: 5 Minutes

Serving: Devour approximately three to 4 ounces within the morning.

Ingredients:

- 1 Apple
- A trickle of pectin (the white part of the citrus. while you peel an orange or lime, that white component you see)
- 1 Big onion

Direction:

1. Mix or blend with water.

Nutrition:

- Calories 138
- Protein 2.1g
- Carbohydrate 35.3g
- Sugar 23.2g
- Fiber 5.7g
- Fat 0.1g

Step 2 Cleanse More to the Organs of the Body

The Viento is blanketed in Dr. Sebi's minor cleaning package deal as it allows you to clean the frame at a mobile stage. You can make your very own Viento system. You can actually but cross instantly to step three.

Step 3 Easy and Stimulate the Blood

The iron will help cleanse the blood, enhance the frame's move, and nourish the cells. As stated, you can purchase or make your very own—it's far very smooth to do that.

Dose: Take the spices as coordinated on the proper framework.

The weight loss plan should be very mild throughout this technique, along with only alkalizing meals, often fruits and greens. Follow Dr. Sebi's nutritional manual. However, some items on the listing should no longer be fed on while trying to reverse extreme health conditions.

Matters on the listing to eat: Culmination, greens together with lettuce, lambs sector, dandelion greens, mustard vegetables, amaranth vegetables and lettuce, mushrooms, vegetables, coconut (water and jelly), natural teas, inexperienced juices, and smoothies.

*Constructing up to Water Fast*

- Start with three days of bowel cleanse.
- Consume a complete plant-based total food regimen for seven days.
- Do another effective 3-day bowel cleanse consuming uncooked culmination and greens for the duration of this period.
- Do a seven days mono-rapid ideally on grapes, mango, melon, or apples.
- Follow up with a 3-day juice fast, mainly inexperienced juices and the juices of citrus culmination.
- Begin your water fast.

Reminder: It's far most famous for lengthy fasting. Tries to go to a fasting health center where you may understand individuals who can help you thru the difficult days beforehand. In case you aren't capable of going to a fasting health facility, it might be vital to have help around you.

*Who Ought not to Fast*

It isn't always recommended that some people go on a water fast. These encompass:

- Pregnant ladies.
- Those are handling anorexia.
- People are laid low with debilitating diseases and have little energy.

- Those in advanced stages of diseases, e.g., Cancers.
- Individuals who are affected by intense intellectual disorders that require professional treatment. If a less severe mental ailment torments you, it's far essential to have support around you.

The fast must be broken successfully.

- Start with the handy juices, vegetable juices, non-sweet fruit juices. Have them for three consecutive days (assuming a 7 to ten days water rapid. The longer the water fasts, the slower and more prolonged the re-feeding length).
- Have natural culmination for some other two days.
- Introduce mild raw salads.
- Slowly introduce other foods.

Note: Eat small food as wished, chunk foods well, pay attention to the frame's signals.

## Via Juicing

After the initial bowel clean of at least three days, have handy juices and teas. This consists of inexperienced or vegetable juices precisely, and you will have more of those at the start, then add fruit juices (citruses and melons).

- Constructing as much as a juice speedy
- Three days of colon cleanse.
- Seven days all-natural culmination and greens.
- Begin juicing.
- Examine constipation.

The duration varies; set a minimum goal of 21 days. Take natural teas, such as those mentioned above, other growth water intake.

Tip: Gracefully taste your juices within the mouth earlier than swallowing.

Vain Water Fasting and Juicing

With this approach, a deliberate sample is created, consuming a balance of fruit juices and water.

- Blended water and juice plan
- Juice in the mornings
- Water within the days
- Juice at nights

## Alternative Methods to Cure Herpes

The more you keep your herpes under control, the less chance you have of suffering from other STDs, worsening symptoms or spreading to a future partner.

However, many people are hesitant to try alternative methods for treating their herpes because of the fear that it will worsen their symptoms and cause them trouble in side effects or contraindications.

Every year, nearly 1/3 of the world's population is infected with HSV-1 or HSV-2. Increasingly, people are looking for alternative treatments to traditional medicine to cure their herpes. However, many of these alternatives may have contraindications or side effects that can cause more harm.

## Acupuncture

Acupuncture has been used for thousands of years, first by the Chinese, and then spread through Eastern countries such as Japan, Taiwan, Korea, Vietnam, and Thailand. It has gained popularity throughout America and other countries thanks to Hollywood stars such as Jennifer Aniston, who have shown support for this practice by endorsing it. It is a type of alternative medicine that uses needles to relieve pain, improve blood circulation, and stimulate the body to feel better overall. It is believed that it will also help specific health conditions such as acne, fatigue, menstrual pain, and many other problems. Acupuncture can treat herpes by stimulating particular acupuncture points on the body, such as the eye area, neck area, or behind the ears. It is believed that with this practice, the person can improve her immune system and fight off the viruses better.

## Herbs

People from different countries have used Asian herbs for many years due to their natural properties that help cure diseases like leukemia and even cancer and HIV. People use herbs to improve the immune system. Herbs have antibacterial, anti-inflammatory, and antioxidant properties that help to cure diseases such as herpes. It is recommended that one take a tea made from powdered roasted ginger, garlic, and ginseng or Chinese Ginseng five times a day for two months and feel the health inside.

A hospital in Thailand has been practicing this technique since eight years ago where patients can get treatment for herpes. The hospital performs acupuncture on their patients who come there with different types of the herpes virus to reduce the duration of the ailment down to three years within 12 months. This hospital also offers healthy food and herbal teas to its patients.

There is also a clinic in the Philippines where they offer free treatment for people affected by this virus and do not have enough money to pay for online or traditional Chinese Medicine. They perform acupuncture on the patient and promote their products to prevent cold sores from coming back.

The person has decided that they want to spend more time with her family and loved ones instead of avoiding them because of her herpes. They would like to teach others who suffer from this disease how to get rid of it naturally without having side effects or contraindications like chemotherapy drugs which can be very dangerous.

The herpes virus is a common sexually transmitted disease, and the person has been struggling with this disease for some time. Traditional medicine has not helped cure the condition, and therefore they find alternative methods to conventional medicine through researching online resources and chatting with friends. The person has found that herbal remedies and acupuncture can help traditional medicine alternatives.

The person hopes that these new alternatives will help her get rid of her herpes once and for all. They also use acupuncture to prevent the herpes virus from causing future cold sores. Acupressure on the back and neck is used for this purpose for them to stay healthy and look beautiful all the time. There is nothing wrong with using these alternatives in this case because they can be very effective in curing herpes.

People from different countries have used Asian herbs for many years due to their natural properties that help cure diseases like leukemia and even cancer and HIV. People use herbs to improve the immune system. Herbs have antibacterial, anti-inflammatory, and antioxidant properties that help to cure diseases such as herpes.

The person has researched online about herbs for herpes and taken precautions to avoid getting this disease again. Herbs such as Aloe Vera, Onion, Cayenne Pepper, Lemongrass Oil, and Coconut Oil can be very effective in curing herpes. These herbs contain antiviral properties which can help the body fight off the virus and stay healthy.

There is also a woman in Indonesia who has experienced firsthand how well acupuncture can cure herpes. They tested the theory herself by trying a new medicine advertised on television that would cure her herpes. However, they did not experience any results until they later tried acupuncture treatment, healing them of their cold sores within ten days. This has convinced them that this treatment is much better than using a simple ointment to treat their herpes.

Many people have been cured of their herpes by using alternative medicines and therapies such as acupuncture and herbal medicine. It is believed that the person will be able to use these alternative forms of treatment to cure herpes faster in the future. However, they must do so with caution as inevitable side effects should be kept in mind, such as bleeding, bruising, numbness after acupuncture, or allergic reactions to herbal medicine. They should also research if these treatments are effective for curing this disease before giving them a try.

## Homemade Remedies Can Be More Effective

If you've tried pharmaceutical medications but never found a good solution for your herpes, alternative medicine can help. That's because herbs and homeopathic remedies are usually natural and work best with the body's healing capabilities.

Most of the time, they are available without a prescription and can be used to complement your treatment for herpes. If traditional treatments alone just aren't enough, then alternative remedies could help you find relief.

Herbal remedies are made from plant and herbal ingredients. They can be 'powdered' or 'liquid' and function by stimulating the immune system. You can combine herbs individually or as part of a daily routine of homeopathic remedies.

This means they work in a similar way to vaccine: This also prevents the virus from spreading from one person to another.

Herbal remedies for herpes don't contain any known side effects and are FDA approved as well. As a result, you can take them without worrying about any contraindications or symptoms.

## Homeopathic Remedy

There are different homeopathic remedies for herpes.

Homeopathic medicines aim to help the body heal itself by adapting to new circumstances or environments. They use alleviating substances that help your body achieve its best potential of health and strength. This allows the body to become stronger to fight off herpes and keep it healthy and functioning well in general. That's why it's essential to choose the correct homeopathic remedy for each unique individual case of herpes.

Mercurius is famous for its ability to prevent latent and active herpes infections. This is also known as Herpeticum in the German language. It is a powerful homeopathic remedy used in different ways, including a liquid form to apply to sore or inflamed areas. Just remember never to use it more than once a day.

Thuja is famous for its effectiveness in battling symptoms such as itchiness, irritation, pain and swelling, and stress and fatigue associated with herpes. This means that using Thuja often boosts your immune system while treating your herpes effectively.

Arnica is a remedy that generally works well in alleviating pain, swelling, redness, and itching. It does so by boosting your body's natural healing abilities to help it get rid of herpes from the virus itself.

Just like homeopathy, herbal and homeopathic remedies can be taken for as long as needed or until your herpes has gone away completely.

Americans are spending a lot of money on treatments for their herpes infections. The treatments that have been proven to work include Valtrex. Some other remedies are more natural and don't have as many side effects.

We will explore what causes these infections, some new treatment methods and how they work, and the best way to prevent a herpes infection in the first place.

To promote safe sex, prevent sexually transmitted diseases (STDs), and promote sexual health, the Ministry of Health has introduced a new program called "HIV/AIDS Prevention and Control in Schools" that aims to provide school children with information about STDs. There is an increasing number of reported cases indicating that HPV mainly genital warts and genital herpes. The Ministry of Health has chosen the campaign "School health promotion for the three STDs; HPV, HSV, and HIV" as its medium to educate young people about STDs.

On July 2, 2011, the Ministry of Health (MoH) released a 'clinical report on genital herpes' and an educational brochure on the condition. The report revealed that 40% of patients with a positive test result for genital herpes never sought medical attention, while 70% were unaware that medication was available to cure it.

The MoH report also stated that one in ten people in Korea is infected with HSV-1 and HSV-2, responsible for causing genital warts and herpes. However, most people do not know they have contracted genital warts or genital herpes and therefore do not seek treatment. One in three men does not even recognize the symptoms of genital warts.

The report stated that 5,502 patients were diagnosed with genital herpes in 2014, increasing 556 cases from the past year.

Although this new program is an excellent first step, it is not enough. It's essential to stress condom use and promote safe sex practices because HPV and HSV can be spread through skin-to-skin contact even when wearing a condom.

Timeline of Vaccines and Drugs Development for HSV in Korea

The list above shows the development timeline of all vaccines and drugs available in Korea. Unfortunately, many of these drugs have serious side effects or cannot eliminate the herpes virus from the body. Perplex is one example. The company that created this drug was fined because FDA didn't approve it. This drug is still being used in Korea and has never been proven to be a safe product.

The following table lists all the vaccines and drugs that have been licensed by the Ministry of Food and Drug Safety.

This new study was performed by Kong Kyun-Jinn, Korea University Ansan Hospital, Kyunggi-do Ansan in Korea. This study found three new compounds related to HSV-2. It is believed that these compounds can reduce HSV symptoms by blocking immune activation through various pathways.

## A Simple Vision Of The Functions Of The Immune System

What Exactly Is the Immune System?

Sickness is caused by bacteria, toxins, or viruses that enter the body, as well as mutating cells within the body. We'd perish quickly if we didn't have any kind of defense against even the most basic elements. Our defense is comprised of a complex network of organs, cells, and tissues that work together to form our Immune System, which first defends against invading bacteria or viruses and then attacks if anything gets through.

There are three types of immunity in your immune system.There are three types of immunity: innate immunity acquired immunity and passive immunity.

These immunities comprise two immunity systems, each of which responds in its way. These are the adaptive and innate immune responses, respectively. Two distinct systems, yet one immune system, interact in complex and critical ways. There can be serious consequences if their balance is off.

The Innate System (Innate Immunity)

Your innate immunity is created by your innate system. That is the immunity you were born with. It is your body's second line of defense, attacking anything that it perceives as a threat. This system is known as nonspecific because it responds to every threat in the same way. It also reacts the same way to every infection. As a result, the innate system is also known as non-adaptive. The following are the components of the non-adaptive system:

- Acidity in the stomach
- White blood cells with phagocytic morphology
- Fever
- Your skin oils contain enzymes.
- Your tears contain enzymes.
- Inflammation
- The cough reflex
- Antimicrobial agents.
- phlegm (traps tiny particles and bacteria)

### System of Adaptation

An acquired immunity is created by the adaptive system. It is the third line of defense for your body. It is not only adaptive but also specific. That is, it can tell the difference between one pathogen and another and responds differently to each one. Although your adaptive immune system may take some time fighting off a pathogen the first time it encounters it, after defending against it once, it learns the pathogen's weaknesses. If your immune system allows it to take hold again, it can quickly eradicate it the next time.

The core components of the adaptive system are lymphocytes, which, as previously stated, are a type of white blood cell. First, your B cells recognize an antigen (a pathogen fragment). The TH cells then release cytokines, which activate the B cells (immune cells). This sets off a chain reaction that results in the production of antibodies to eradicate the pathogen. When the crisis is over, your body converts a small portion of the activated B and TH cells into memory cells, which immunize you against the pathogen.

### The passive immunity

Passive immunity is created when antibodies produced outside of the body are used to build immunity. Passive immunity includes the immunity that a baby receives from antibodies in breastmilk. Another type of passive immunity is obtained through immunization (antiserum injection), such as the tetanus antitoxin. Unfortunately, while passive immunity provides immediate protection, it must be repeated. The effects fade after a while.

How Does the Immune System Work?

Your immune system is constantly on the lookout for antigens as you go about your day. Antigens are any foreign invaders that the body recognizes as dangerous. These microorganisms can be viruses, bacteria, or fungi. An antigen can be a chemical, a toxin, a drug, or even an eyelash. They can be proteins (or something else) on the surface of the cells. But that isn't the only thing your immune system needs to be on the lookout for. In your bloodstream, there are also damaged cells called free radicals that steal electrons from healthy cells, damaging them and possibly leading to cancer.

Your body, on the other hand, contains antigens known as HLA antigens that are supposed to be present. These are proteins that occur naturally in your cells. Your immune system recognizes those antigens as harmless and ignores them. So, here's the deal:

How does it know what to attack and what to ignore?

Our bodies are incredible. To begin, unhealthy cells emit "danger" cues to signal their presence. These are referred to as danger-associated molecular patterns (DAMPs). When your immune system recognizes a DAMP, which comes in a variety of forms, it knows which cell to attack and how to attack it. And, because unhealthy cells can be caused by a variety of factors ranging from sunburn to infection to cancer, your body has its work cut out for it.

Aside from that, contact with infectious microbes, or pathogens, triggers an entirely different set of signals. Bacteria and viruses are examples of infectious microbes. Pathogen-associated molecular patterns are the name given to these signals (PAMPs). Each PAMP elicits a distinct response. Allergens such as fungi, pollen, and foods must also be dealt with by the immune system. What your body does in response to each of these It determines how much of an invader that particular allergen is to your body. That is why some people have almost no allergies at all.

What happens after your body recognizes what's familiar and what's foreign?

What Exactly Is an Immune Response?

The immune response is your body's reaction to antigens in your system. When a healthy immune system is attacked, it immediately goes into action, fighting the virus, bacteria, or fungi. If it can't be triggered when it's needed or doesn't have enough resources to eliminate the foreign intruder, it can lead to problems like infection and sickness. However, when the immune system is triggered without cause or refuses to "shut down" after the danger has passed, you can develop autoimmune disease and allergic reactions.

The fact that a healthy immune system is so extensive contributes to its effectiveness. It makes use of nearly every part of the body.

## Skin

Your skin is, as always, your first line of defense. It's similar to the castle's wall and mote. Your skin cells defend themselves against bacteria, viruses, and other microbes by secreting antimicrobial proteins that attack the microbes when they come into contact with them. Immune cells are also formed within the various layers of skin.

## Bone Marrow

Despite their differences, all immune cells begin their lives as stem cells in the bone marrow. They then travel to their final destination. They then mature into the required immune cells. Even though they are derived from the same source, these mature cells can perform the immune function for that part of the body.

The myeloid progenitor stem cell develops into innate immune cells, which fight infection. The lymphoid progenitor stem cell gives rise to adaptive immune cells (B cells and T cells), which fight specific viruses and bacteria. Natural killer cells (NK cells) develop from lymphoid progenitor cells as well. NK cells can function as both adaptive and innate immune cells.

## Bloodstream

Immune cells are constantly patrolling the bloodstream, ready to strike at the first sign of trouble. White blood cells, or leukocytes, are immune cells found in your bloodstream. Doctors can check neutrophils, a type of leukocyte, to see if a bacterial infection has activated your immune system.

Leukocytes are classified into two types: phagocytes and lymphocytes. Lymphocytes write invading pathogen information into the cell so it can be remembered and then eradicates, whereas Phagocytes beat up on the pathogens and destroy what they can.

These two families are made up of five different types of leukocytes, all of which perform an immune function.

Neutrophils, as previously mentioned, are the first immune defense to arrive on the scene in response to microbial infection.

Monocytes are also among the first immune cells to respond to microbial infection.

Basophils are the first immune cells to respond to inflammation. When activated, they release the chemicals heparin and histamine.

B lymphocytes (B cells) and T lymphocytes are examples of lymphocytes (T cells). In the presence of viruses and bacteria, B cells and T cells join forces to initiate a chain reaction that results in the production of antibodies. Cytotoxic T cells and natural killer cells (NK cells) work together to eliminate virus-infected cells.

*Relative Proportions of White Blood Cells in a Healthy Human Body*

| Neutrophils | 60-70% |
| --- | --- |
| Monocytes | 1-6% |
| Eosinophils | 1-3% |
| Basophils | Less than 1% |
| Lymphocytes | 20-30% |

## Antibodies

Lymphocytes produce antibodies, which can then recognize infected or damaged cells and tag them for elimination. However, it is incapable of destroying. That is the function of the NK cells.

Antibodies also fight toxins (both pathological and biological) and activate the complement system, a group of proteins that aid in the elimination of viruses, bacteria, and infected cells.

## Complement

The complement system is made up of more than thirty different proteins that work together to eliminate antigens, specifically infectious microorganisms. The liver is in charge of producing the vast majority of the complement system. These proteins circulate throughout the body via extracellular fluid and blood until they are required.

The immune system then, and only then, sends two signals. Molecules embedded in the microorganism trigger one signal.

Antibodies bound to the microorganism's surface activate the other signal. When one complement is triggered, the next two complements in the sequence are triggered as well. As a result, they create two pathways, both of which lead to the same pivotal protein. When the pathways cross, the pivotal protein is activated, resulting in a gruesome attack on the microorganism.

## Lymphatic System

It has a significant impact on the immune system. The lymphatic system is a network of lymphatic vessels, lymphoid organs, extracellular fluid, and lymph. It is one of the primary routes for bloodstream-to-tissue communication.

The lymphatic vessels run throughout the body and transport waste products. They also contain tissue fluid and immune cells, which make their home in the lymph organs.

Immune cells use this highway to conduct reconnaissance. As the lymphatic system transports the waste products of other cells, immune cells scan it for PAMPs and DAMPs. If something is discovered, the immune response in the cell is activated. It will multiply, and cells will leave in large numbers to crush, kill, and destroy.

## Lymph Nodes

Several small "pathogen traps" can be found along this highway of lymphatic vessels, lymph, and immune cells. These "traps" are called lymph nodes, and they are designed specifically for trapping and eradicating pathogens and other invaders or damaged cells as they pass through. The lymph nodes are simply bean-shaped clusters of immune cells densely packed with white blood cells—every "invader's" worst nightmare.

## Thymus

T cells are immune cells found in the thymus. Your thymus is one of the smaller organs in your upper chest, near your thyroid.

## Spleen

Though the spleen is not directly connected to the lymphatic system, it performs the same basic function, entitling it to be considered a part of it. It is an important part of the body's defenses because it filters the blood and sends the information it gathers. The spleen is also densely packed with immune system cells that are ready to activate and attack the moment a blood-borne pathogen is identified.

## Mucosal Tissue

Mucosal surfaces, which include the lips, ears, nostrils, genital area, eyelids, and anus, are one of the easiest entry points for any virus or bacteria. That is taken care of by our immune system. Mucosal tissue lines our respiratory, digestive, and reproductive tracts. This tissue is responsible for keeping the insides in and the outsides out. But what prevents viruses and bacteria from crossing that line? That's your handy mucosal tissue, which not only acts as a barrier but also has cells on standby. Different areas of the gut also have access areas where immune cells check the contents of the gastrointestinal tract for cause for alarm.

## Inflammation

The inflammatory response is triggered when your tissues are damaged by trauma, bacteria, heat, toxins, or any type of antigen. As a result, your body produces a wide range of chemicals. Prostaglandins, histamine, and bradykinin are a few examples. When these chemicals enter your system, your blood vessels start to leak into the damaged tissues. This causes swelling around the antigen, which helps to isolate it from the rest of your tissues.

The chemicals released during an inflammatory response attract phagocytes, which kill germs and "eat" damaged or dead cells. Phagocytosis is the name given to this process.

What Exactly Is a Modified Immune Response?

Your immune system can respond in one of three ways: efficiently, inadequately, or overly. You have an efficient immune response if your immune system is healthy and adequately protecting you.

If your immune system allows diseases to develop, it is ineffective. An inefficient immune system is typically caused by an immune deficiency disease, unless it is caused by an external source, such as medication. An immune deficiency disease can be primary, meaning you were born with it or acquired, meaning it was caused by another illness.

In addition, the immune system is overactive. Your immune system may become overactive as a result of an allergic reaction or hypersensitivity. When your immune system begins to attack your body, an autoimmune disease can develop. Immune responses are altered in both an inefficient and overactive immune system.

What Causes Your Immune System to Attack Your Body?

Paul Ehrlich proposed the possibility of autoimmune tissue attacks until the turn of the twentieth century. He did not, however, believe that the autoimmune response could become pathological. The 1950s marked the beginning of our understanding of autoimmune diseases and autoantibodies as we know them today.

We've come a long way, but doctors still don't have an answer. They have discovered, however, that certain autoimmune diseases are more common in certain groups of people.

According to a 2014 study published on sciencedirect.com, two women out of everyone man develop an autoimmune disease. Autoimmune diseases typically manifest between the ages of 15 and 44.

They usually prefer one ethnic group over another. Lupus, for example, is more common in Hispanics and African Americans than in Caucasians. Some autoimmune diseases are inherited. For example, if one member of the family has Lupus or multiple sclerosis, the other members are at risk of developing an autoimmune disease. Possibly it won't be the same.

Researchers believe that if you are exposed to certain solvents, chemicals, or environmental factors, you are more likely to develop an autoimmune disease.

Lisa A. Reynolds, Leah T. Stiemsma, B. Brett Finlay, and Stuart E. Turvey hypothesized in 2015 that a lack of germ exposure could lead to an overreactive response to harmless antigens.

A high-sugar, high-fat diet, as well as many processed foods, are thought to cause inflammation, which sets off an autoimmune response and increases the risk of developing an autoimmune disease. As a result, the scope of this book.

A strong immune system is essential for a healthy body. When the immune system is out of balance, it not only fails to defend against antigens, but it can also start attacking itself, resulting in an autoimmune disease that can be fatal. The immune system becomes sensitive to life itself at this point. Simple things like strenuous exercise, the stress of personal problems, travel, and even a simple diet change can all hurt your overall health. Aside from that, even low-level inflammation can increase the risk of developing other diseases such as cardiovascular disease and cancer over time.

# AUTOIMMUNE DISEASES

The field of autoimmunity is still in its infancy in the medical world.

Autoimmunity was first mentioned in history by the German biologist and pathologist Paul Ehrlich, who won the Nobel Prize in Medicine in 1908. Ehrlich coined the term horror autotoxicus (fear of self-poisoning) around the turn of the last century to describe the phenomenon that could occur when a person's defenses turned against him or her. At the time, horror autotoxicus was primarily a clinical observation based on findings in specific patients. Ehrlich was heavily involved in the description of antigens and their chemical structure, as well as the investigation of a new concept known as antitoxins.

He realized that an antigen, as a foreign matter, could be a part of our tissues but be recognized as such by the immune system. In short, he proposed the now-accepted theory that our immune systems can react to something native to our bodies as well as seek out strangers. He had no idea how or what to do.

Around the same time, Ehrlich's contemporary, the great internist William Osler, studied skin diseases that he thought were related to tuberculosis (TB) but were autoimmune diseases. Although he eventually concluded that these diseases were distinct from tuberculosis, he lacked the tools to prove their biological origins. Because antibodies were not discovered until the 1950s, all of these researchers fantasized about what "might be," which is essentially the same process that all medical researchers use today.

A decade later, in the 1960s, when doctors Gerald Edelman of Rockefeller University and Rodney Peters of Oxford University defined the structure of an antibody, the concept of autoimmunity as a cause of human illness became medical lore. This resulted in the development of laboratory tests to aid in the diagnosis of autoimmune diseases. T and B cells were discovered soon after. The discovery of the origins of antibodies and autoreactive cells catapulted autoimmunity into the forefront of science and medicine research. Given that all of this occurred in the last forty years, we have made incredible progress.

The human immune system gathers chemicals and cells that fight and protect our bodies from infections caused by bacteria and viruses. As a result, the immune system is critical in protecting us from microbial infections. In autoimmune disorders, the immune system malfunctions and misidentifies the body's cells and tissues as foreign invaders and begins killing them. What happens when the immune system is unable to distinguish between its cells and foreign invaders? When this happens, the affected body produces auto-antibodies, which attack the body's cells by mistake. On the other hand, regulatory T cells fail to perform their function of keeping the immune system in check. As a result, your body's cells are mistakenly attacked.

Autoimmune disorders are broadly classified into two types: Autoimmune disorders affecting specific organs. The disorder primarily affects one organ, whereas the other is a non-organ-specific autoimmune disorder that can affect multiple organs and systems. There are approximately 80 autoimmune disorders, with severity ranging from minor to disabling, depending on the affected organ and degree of disability.

Autoimmune diseases are extremely common, affecting over 23.5 million people in the United States alone. Autoimmune disorders are a major cause of disability and death. As we all know, there are many (approximately 80) autoimmune disorders, some of which are extremely common, while others are extremely rare.

## What Exactly Is an Autoimmune Disease?

You approach the person to say "hello," tap them on the shoulder, and when they turn around, you realize you've never met this person before. They are an outsider. You have that panicked moment where you try to think of something to say, and then the awkward explanations begin.

Autoimmune diseases are very similar to this illustration. To protect itself from germs and viruses, our body has developed an intricate and amazing security system: our immune system. The diligent security guards. White blood cells are part of this system. They patrol the vascular system, which is the body's highway system. The vascular system is a network of veins and arteries that transport blood from the heart to the rest of the body and back again. They patrol the vascular system, looking for invading organisms such as viruses and germs. When the white blood cells come across these "bad" cells floating around, they attack them. When a person has an autoimmune disease, the white blood cells misinterpret their cells and mistake them for harmful, invading cells. As a result, white cells swarm and attack those cells. White cells can be misled by any of our cells, organs, or systems. Your white cells will continue to attack these cells once they have been identified as dangerous.

## A Neutrophil Antibody in Close-up (white blood cell)

You have an autoimmune disease if this happens. More than eighty different types of autoimmune diseases have been identified, affecting over 23 million Americans. Women account for 80 percent of those diagnosed. Each autoimmune disease is associated with a distinct system, organ, or cell that white blood cells have misidentified as a dangerous foreign body.

Are women simply weaker and more susceptible to disease?

The exact opposite is true. Women have two X chromosomes. The X chromosome contains over 1000 different types of genes. The Y chromosome, on the other hand, has just over 100 genes. That is if one of their X chromosomes has a defective gene, a female's redundant gene on the other X chromosome can step in and replace the defective gene. It makes females less susceptible to X gene-linked hereditary diseases and infectious diseases, and it causes them to live statistically longer and healthier lives than men. In the case of autoimmune diseases, however, the XX chromosomes are the problem.

The immune system genes are found on the X chromosome. So, why do women suffer from autoimmune diseases? Isn't having a stronger immune system a good thing? No, it does not. The only chromosome that is not doubled in both men and women is the X chromosome. To prevent a woman from having two copies of the X chromosome's genes, her body naturally shuts down (inactivates) the redundant genes on the chromosome. The body is intelligent enough to do this inactivation in a pattern (usually 50/50 per X chromosome). However, it occasionally fails to turn off a redundant gene. Or it will use the redundant genes in an inefficient manner (60/40 or 80/20). The body unusually inactivates the genes. It's known as "skewed gene inactivation." When it comes to autoimmune diseases, women's biology works against them. However, researchers and doctors are unsure why female hormones frequently appear to trigger autoimmune diseases in some way. It is normal for autoimmune disease symptoms to appear during puberty.

These are some of the warning signs:

- Inflammation of the Joints
- Joint Discomfort
- Pain in the abdomen
- Chronic Diarrhea or Constipation
- Glands that are swollen
- Other Long-Term Digestive Problems
- Flu-like Symptoms
- Having difficulty swallowing food or beverages
- Weight Gain or Loss That Isn't Explained
- Rashes on the skin or other skin problems
- Chronic Fatigue or Exhaustion

Please consult your doctor if you are experiencing any of these symptoms.

## Treatment and Cause

Many people complain that getting an autoimmune disease diagnosis is difficult. Unfortunately, this is sometimes true for a variety of reasons. Diagnosis of an autoimmune disease is not a simple process. Most of these diseases do not have a specific blood test that can tell you whether you have them or not. Rather, it is a process of looking for markers in the blood, noting symptoms, and, in some cases, taking tissue samples. It can also be complicated because many of the symptoms are caused by other illnesses or viruses. It can take some time and patience to get the right diagnosis. I've discovered that having the right doctor is critical. My rheumatologist was able to diagnose me after my other doctors were unable to.

The causes of autoimmune diseases are unknown to doctors and researchers. They do, however, have a list of things they know are contributing factors or commonalities among patients.

These are the items:

- Genetics
- Lifestyle
- Environmental Aspects
- Stress
- Weight
- Diet
- Smoking

Autoimmune diseases can have a wide range of severity in terms of how they affect the person suffering from them. One person's life may be relatively unaffected, whereas the next person's life may be severely impacted. The severity of the disease is a factor in many of these cases.Concerns about lifestyle and the environment Smoking and being overweight both have a statistically significant negative impact on disease progression. Furthermore, someone with a strong genetic link appears to have gotten the short end of the stick when it comes to the severity of the disease.

Autoimmune Disease Diagnosis

Assume that these diseases appear to be difficult to define. In that case, they are even more difficult to diagnose, as anyone with an autoimmune disease can attest.

As you will see in the following chapters, it is not nearly that simple with autoimmune diseases. We take a history and conduct a physical examination, but then the problems start.

Because there are no definitive diagnostic laboratory tests for autoimmune disease, it is extremely difficult to diagnose. Yes, antibodies can be produced in a blood test on a patient with suspected autoimmune disease.

We might even find an autoantibody. However, it is not a guarantee that the patient has the disease. T and B cells that are autoreactive are not specific because they can occur in healthy people. So, when an autoimmune disease is suspected, laboratory tests simply confirm what the doctor already suspects. Clinical training and the doctor's clinical impression are what generate the diagnosis, which is why it is critical to find a well-trained specialist.

Aside from clinical difficulties, many other factors contribute to the difficulty of diagnosing autoimmune disease:

- Symptoms can creep into a woman's life so gradually that the changes are misattributed to aging or stress.
- Even within the same person, symptoms are not consistent.
- When autoimmune diseases arise, because they are initially specific to a specific organ, the patient is usually referred to the (apparently) appropriate medical specialist.

For example, a patient with glandular problems may be referred to an endocrinologist by her internist. A hematologist may be summoned to evaluate the diseases of the blood, and anyone experiencing neurological symptoms will be rushed to a neurologist. When autoimmune-related symptoms first appear, the rheumatologist (who specializes in autoimmune diseases) is often the last specialist to be considered.

Because their symptoms—fatigue and pain, for example—are immeasurable and nonspecific, physicians unfamiliar with autoimmune diseases frequently send patients away undiagnosed (or refer them to a psychiatrist or put them on tranquilizers). This is especially true for fibromyalgia and chronic fatigue syndrome (CFS), which may be symptoms of an autoimmune disease but are not classified as such.

One of the reasons that fibromyalgia and CFS, among other diseases, are not currently considered autoimmune diseases is that no autoantibody has been identified in these conditions. There has been no evidence of a chemical change or a change in a cell population. Autoimmune diseases are frequently associated with other autoimmune diseases, and second, I am convinced that they are real and not the result of a psychological anomaly. I do not doubt that these diseases will provide important clues to the immune system's many other diseases in the future. I'm also convinced that if we find the right antigens for the antibodies, some of them could be autoimmune diseases.

Aside from playing subway detective, there is no substitute for sitting down with a patient and taking her history. When a patient walks into my office, I begin my diagnosis. If she walks in confidently, I notice how strong her grip is when she shakes my hand. Is she by herself or with a relative? Is she looking at you with hope or despair? I try to decide whether she wants all of the facts or just a summary if she understands what I'm saying.

You must inquire about everything:

- Are you a good artist?
- Are you going gray too soon?
- Are you afflicted with any birthmarks?
- Are you left-handed or right-handed?

Everything is important.

It is well known that people with autoimmune diseases have a higher incidence of left handedness. These people are talented artists, excellent mathematicians, and have excellent hand-eye coordination. For example, when I look at a young girl who pitches for a Little League team, I notice that she is almost always left-handed or ambidextrous. Not long ago, I went to a game where a little girl was pitching against my son, who was batting. She could catch with either hand and pitched lefty. I was sitting next to her mother at the time and said, " "Oh my goodness, your daughter is gifted. Has she always been this way?"

## Corticosteroids

Corticosteroids (also known as steroids) are synthetic medications that mimic the hormone cortisol, which your body naturally produces. These medications are used to reduce inflammation (the body's process of attacking foreign or dangerous cells in the body) and to reduce immune system activity by knocking someone's immune system back with an autoimmune disease. It does, however, leave the person with a weakened immune system. Prednisone and cortisone are two of the most commonly prescribed corticosteroids.

## Immunosuppressants

Immunosuppressants are medications that are prescribed to suppress the immune system, as the name implies. They are used to treat a variety of conditions, including autoimmune diseases and anti-rejection medications for organ transplants. Immunosuppressants come in a variety of forms (including corticosteroids). What is prescribed is determined by your disease and the tolerance of your body. Immunosuppressants come in a variety of forms, including:

- Corticosteroids
- prednisone
- prednisolone
- Inhibitors of Janus kinase
- tofacitinib
- Inhibitors of calcineurin
- mTOR inhibitors

- Cyclosporine
- IMDH inhibitors
- sirolimus
- methotrexate
- leflunomide
- Biologics
- adalimumab
- certolizumab
- etanercept
- infliximab
- rituximab
- Monoclonal antibodies
- Basiliximab

This is far from a comprehensive list of the medications available. Rather, it is a synopsis. Doctors frequently prescribe dietary changes as well as lifestyle changes.

## Autoimmune Disease Types

This section will include a brief overview of the most common autoimmune diseases, as well as information on each one. This is not a method of diagnosing a disease; only a qualified doctor can do so. That is basic information that can help you identify potential disease symptoms and encourage you to consult with a qualified doctor.

## Celiac disease

Celiac disease is an autoimmune disorder that causes a person to be unable to consume gluten. When you consume gluten, your body responds with an autoimmune reaction that damages your small intestine.

## Crohn's Disease

Crohn's disease is an autoimmune disease of the bowels. It causes inflammation of the gastrointestinal tract's lining and walls. It is a very painful disease, but it is not usually fatal.

## Eosinophilic esophagitis (EoE)

Eosinophilic esophagitis is a food allergy-related autoimmune disease. It causes esophageal inflammation and the growth of eosinophilic cells, a type of white blood cell that is specific to the esophagus. When these cells proliferate excessively, they cause swelling and other autoimmune reactions.

## Fibromyalgia

Fibromyalgia is characterized by widespread pain, tenderness, insomnia, and exhaustion. It is not classified as an autoimmune disease, but it is associated with a number of them. Fibromyalgia has also been linked to the development or exacerbation of depression.

## Graves' syndrome

Graves' disease is an autoimmune disorder affecting the thyroid gland. It causes the gland to produce an excessive amount of hormone. It causes heat intolerance, nervousness, and weight loss. Women are affected at a much higher rate than men.

## Lupus

Lupus is an autoimmune disease that causes inflammation in a variety of body systems. Lupus is classified into three types: Systemic Lupus Erythematosus (SLE), Discoid Lupus, and Drug-Induced Lupus are all types of lupus. Lyme disease Lyme disease is an autoimmune disease caused by a deer tick bite.

## Multiple sclerosis (MS) (MS)

MS is an autoimmune disease that affects the brain and spinal cord. The autoimmune reaction occurs when the body attacks the myelin sheathing of the nerves, slowing the transmission of messages from the brain to other parts of the body.

## Psoriasis

Psoriasis is an autoimmune skin disease. The autoimmune response results in red scaly patches caused by excessive skin cell production.

## Diabetes type 1

Type 1 diabetes is an autoimmune disease in which the pancreas fails to produce enough insulin. Insulin is a hormone that aids in the transport of blood sugar into cells. Without insulin, glucose builds up in the body, causing coma and even death.

## Autoimmune Disorders Diagnosis

An autoimmune disease is notoriously difficult to diagnose, especially in its early stages. Autoimmune diseases that affect multiple organs and systems are extremely difficult to diagnose.

Diagnostic methods can vary depending on the type of autoimmune disorder:

- X-rays
- Biopsy
- Certain blood tests, including those that detect autoantibodies, are available.
- Examination of the body
- History of the patient
- Test for Antinuclear Antibodies
- Electrophoresis of Proteins
- C Complementary Test
- C Protein Reactive Test

## Autoimmune Inflammatory Diseases That Are Common

### HEPATITIS AUTOIMMUNE

Autoimmune hepatitis is a long-term and chronic disease in which the body's immune cells mistakenly attack normal liver cells and components, resulting in liver damage and inflammation. Autoimmune hepatitis is a serious condition that, if left untreated, can worsen and become more severe over time. If this condition worsens, it can lead to liver failure or cirrhosis. Cirrhosis develops when scar tissue replaces normal liver cells and tissue, obstructing normal blood flow through the liver. When the liver fails to function properly, it results in liver failure.

### COMMON SOURCES OF AUTOIMMUNE DISEASE

Environmental factors, genetic predisposition, autoimmunity, or a combination of these factors may all contribute to autoimmune hepatitis.

Who is More Likely to Develop This Autoimmune Disorder?

This chronic disorder can affect people of any age or ethnicity. However, this disorder is more common in women.

### AUTOIMMUNE HEPATITIS TYPES

There are several kinds of autoimmune hepatitis. Type 1 autoimmune hepatitis can strike at any age or stage, but it is more common in North America and primarily affects adolescents and young adults. Females account for roughly 70% of those affected by this autoimmune disorder.

- People with autoimmune hepatitis may also have:
- Graves' disease,
- Crohn's disease,
- Celiac disease,
- Proliferative glomerulonephritis,
- Sjogren's syndrome,
- Rheumatoid arthritis,
- Ulcerative colitis,
- Systemic Lupus,
- Type 1 diabetes, and other autoimmune diseases.
- Type 2 autoimmune hepatitis is less common than type 1 and mostly affects children. People with type 2 autoimmune hepatitis can have any of the disorders listed above.

### AUTOIMMUNE HEPATITIS SYMPTOMS

- Yellowish skin or jaundice
- Urine that is dark in color and stool that is light in color
- Joint discomfort
- Fatigue
- Nausea

- Pain in the liver
- Reduced or complete loss of appetite
- Rashes on the skin

Autoimmune hepatitis symptoms can range from mild to severe. When a healthcare professional diagnoses the disease, some people may have mild flu symptoms, while others may not have any visible symptoms. However, symptoms of the disease can appear later in life.

## AUTOIMMUNE HEPATITIS DIAGNOSIS

A health professional can diagnose the disease based on a physical examination, the patient's history, blood tests, and a liver biopsy.

## TREATMENT OPTIONS FOR AUTOIMMUNE HEPATITIS

Patients with autoimmune hepatitis who have few to mild symptoms may or may not require medical treatment. Based on medical examinations and the patient's history, a health care provider can make a more informed treatment decision. This disorder may go into remission in people who have the disease but only have mild symptoms. Remission is a brief period during which the patient is symptom-free and his blood tests and liver biopsy show an improvement in liver function.

## CORTICOSTEROIDS

Corticosteroids are medications that reduce swelling and suppress immune system activity. Corticosteroids (usually prednisone) are prescribed by doctors to treat both types of autoimmune hepatitis. Patients are given a high dose at first, which is gradually reduced as symptoms improve.

## IMMUNOSUPPRESSANTS

Drugs that suppress immune system activity prevent the immune system from producing autoantibodies and prevent the autoimmune response that causes inflammation. Azathioprine is the most commonly used drug in this class, along with prednisone, to treat this fatal disorder.

Because these drugs have some mild to severe side effects, health care professionals must closely monitor patients and adjust the dose as needed.

## TRANSPLANTATION OF THE LIVER

When autoimmune hepatitis progresses to end-stage liver failure or cirrhosis, a liver transplant is required. It is a very complicated and costly treatment method. The surgery is usually successful, and the patient is advised to take prescription medications for an extended period to prevent transplant rejections and other infections.

## AUTOIMMUNE HEPATITIS COMPLICATIONS

People who have autoimmune hepatitis are more likely to develop liver cancer. A health professional uses a liver ultrasound to continuously monitor the patient. Ultrasound examinations are performed by specialized and trained technicians or doctors. Ultrasound images of the liver can reveal information about liver cancer or cancerous tissues in the liver.

## RHEUMATOID ARTHRITIS (RA)

Rheumatoid arthritis is an autoimmune, chronic, long-lasting, disabling, progressive, and inflammatory disease that causes joint pain and inflammation in the tissues surrounding the joints; it may also affect other body organs. This disease primarily affects the hands and feet, but it can affect any joint in the human body. The most common complaints from rheumatoid patients are stiff joints, tiredness, and a general sense of being ill.

People with this autoimmune disorder produce autoantibodies in their blood, which misinterpret their body tissues as foreign invaders and attack and kill them, causing inflammation. Rheumatoid arthritis patients' immune systems attack the lining of their joints, causing them to become inflamed. Rheumatoid arthritis, unlike osteoarthritis, does not cause wear and tear damage. Instead, it attacks and destroys the lining of the joints, causing a painful swelling that can lead to bone deformity and bone erosion. Rheumatoid arthritis, if left untreated, can cause permanent joint damage.

Rheumatoid arthritis is a disease that affects the entire body. It primarily affects the joints, but patients may also experience fever and fatigue. Rheumatoid arthritis patients are at a higher risk of having a heart attack than the general population.

According to the John Hopkins Arthritis Center in the United States:

- Rheumatoid arthritis affects about 1-2 percent of the world's population.
- Rheumatoid arthritis becomes more common as people get older. This disorder affects about 5% of women over the age of 55.
- In the United States, approximately 70 people out of every 100,000 are affected.
- Smokers are four times more likely than nonsmokers to develop rheumatoid arthritis.
- Rheumatoid arthritis outnumbers multiple sclerosis and leukemia in terms of prevalence. Unfortunately, the severity of its effects and awareness are more limited to patients, their relatives, and caregivers because the general public is unaware of this disabling disorder.
- Symptoms of the disease do not always remain active; they come and go. At some point, the symptoms may become minor.They can be extremely painful and severe at times. A patient may experience an unexpected outbreak of the disease.
- Although there is no known cure for this disease, early detection and treatment may slow the disease's progression and make symptoms less severe and easier to manage.

## SYMPTOMS AND SIGNS

We hear and read these words all the time. What's the distinction between a sign and a symptom? It's quite simple. A symptom is something that a patient feels and experiences, whereas a sign is something that other people can see as a doctor. In rheumatoid arthritis, for example, joint pain is a symptom, and inflammation is a sign.

Rheumatoid arthritis, as we all know, is a chronic and debilitating disease. Different people may experience this disorder in different ways and may have different symptoms. Some patients' symptoms may come and go, whereas others may have them all the time. A patient who has a sudden severe onset of this disorder may go to bed healthy but wake up the next morning with severe rheumatoid pain and may be unable to get out of bed.

Rheumatoid arthritis usually begins quietly. The disease's signs and symptoms appear gradually over weeks or months.

Initially, the patient may feel pain and stiffness in one joint, which is usually accompanied by severe pain when moving that joint. Rheumatoid pain is typically felt in small joints at first, such as the toes and fingers. The number of affected joints varies from case to case, but they all affect at least five joints at the same time. Rheumatoid arthritis is a polyarthritis disease, which means it affects an increasing number of joints over time.

Joints That Are Frequently Affected

THE FINGER'S BASIC AND MIDDLE JOINTS

- Ankles
- Knee
- Elbow Shoulders

Symptoms that do not have a specific cause may appear months before the other symptoms.

- Fever of low intensity
- Depression
- Fatigue Malaise

Symptoms that are no longer present.

Symptoms of this autoinflammatory disease are not consistent and can appear and disappear at any time. The patient may experience few symptoms for months, and then experience a sudden outbreak of the symptoms.

RISK FACTORS

What exactly is a risk factor for a disease? A risk factor is anything that increases the likelihood of developing a disease or condition. Cigarette smoking, for example, raises the risk of developing lung cancer, and obesity raises the risk of type 2 diabetes.

The main risk factors for rheumatoid arthritis are as follows:

- Hormones

Certain hormones are implicated in the onset of rheumatoid arthritis. Males with low testosterone levels are more likely to develop rheumatoid arthritis in the future.

- Age

Although anyone of any age can develop this disease, people between the ages of 40 and 60 are at a higher risk than others.

- Biology

Although rheumatoid arthritis is not a hereditary disease, some people are predisposed to develop it due to a genetic mutation. People who have a close family member with rheumatoid arthritis are more likely to develop the disease.

- Gender

Rheumatoid arthritis affects women two to three times more than men, according to the Mayo Clinic. This could be due to the hormone estrogen. However, because it is still a theory, it must be proven.

- Cigarette smoking

Smoking is associated with an increased risk of developing rheumatoid arthritis, so smokers are at a higher risk.

## CAUSES

Rheumatoid arthritis develops when the immune system mistakenly attacks the lining of the joint membranes (also known as synovium). As a result of this synovium destruction, the inflammation thickens the synovium, which can eventually destroy the bone and cartilage in the joints. Ligaments and tendons weaken and stretch, causing the joint to deform and lose alignment and shape. Nobody knows what causes this process to begin, but genetics is thought to play a role.

Although inherited genes do not cause rheumatoid arthritis, they can increase a person's susceptibility to it.

## RHEUMATOID ARTHRITIS COMPLICATIONS

- Enhanced Risk of Lung Disease

Because rheumatoid arthritis is an inflammatory disease, people who have it are more likely to develop lung inflammation and scarring, resulting in shortness of breath.

- Osteoporosis

Rheumatoid arthritis and the medications used to treat it can increase the risk of developing osteoporosis.

- Increased Risk of Cardiovascular Disease

Rheumatoid arthritis can cause artery hardening and blockage in the heart. It may also increase the likelihood of inflammation of the sac that surrounds the heart.

Carpal Tunnel Syndrome (CTS)

Carpal tunnel syndrome can be exacerbated by rheumatoid arthritis.

## RHEUMATOID ARTHRITIS DIAGNOSIS

This disease is extremely difficult to diagnose in its early stages. Its main signs and symptoms (stiffness and inflammation) are similar to those of many other conditions. A doctor will perform a physical examination to determine whether or not a patient has the disease. The doctor will examine the joints to determine whether they are inflamed or not, as well as their movability. The patient will be questioned about his or her symptoms. For an accurate diagnosis, the patient should inform the doctor of all signs and symptoms.

## Blood tests for diagnosis

BLOOD TEST DIAGNOSIS

- ESR
- Anemia blood test
- Protein C reactive
- Test for Rheumatoid Factor
- MRI scans
- X-rays, and image scans

How Can You Tell If You Have Rheumatoid Arthritis?

It is critical to distinguish rheumatoid arthritis from other conditions that can cause joint pain, such as:

- Arthritis caused by gonococci
- Sarcoidosis
- Whipple's disease
- Rheumatic fever (acute)

To stay away from it, The American College of Rheumatology established the classification criteria for rheumatoid arthritis in 1987. Six warning signs that you should be aware of if you are concerned about suffering from it are as follows:

1. Radiological findings suggest possible joint erosion.
2. Morning stiffness that lasts more than an hour for the past six weeks
3. Arthritis and soft tissue swelling must be present in at least three of the fourteen joints/joint groups for at least six weeks.
4. The rheumatoid factor must be higher than the 95th percentile.
5. Subcutaneous nodules should be found in specific locations.
6. Symmetric arthritis should be present for at least six weeks.

At least four of the above conditions must be present to confirm the presence of rheumatoid arthritis. Initially, these criteria were intended for research rather than diagnosis. If the doctor waits to meet all of the American College of Rheumatology criteria, the condition may worsen.

## Rheumatoid Arthritis Treatment Options

Unfortunately, there is no cure for rheumatoid arthritis at this time. The treatment options aim to reduce inflammation, pain in the joints, slow joint deformation, or limit disability. A physiotherapist and an occupational therapist can advise patients on how to protect their joints. Surgery may be required depending on the time of diagnosis (whether the disease was detected at an early stage or not) and the extent of the damage.

*The most commonly used drugs*

- Corticosteroids
- Nonsteroidal anti-inflammatory drugs (NSAIDs)
- Disease-modifying anti-rheumatic drugs
- Immunosuppressants
- Occupational therapy
- Surgery
- Lifestyle changes (such as acupuncture, massage, electrotherapy, and so on)

## Lupus

Lupus is an autoimmune inflammatory disease in which the body's immune system becomes overactive and begins killing healthy and normal tissues by mistake. As a result, symptoms such as swelling, inflammation, and damage to the lungs, kidneys, heart, skin, and joints begin to appear in those who are affected.

## Lupus Comes in Several Varieties

### LUPUS ERYTHEMATOSUS DISCOID

This type of Lupus affects only the skin. It is distinguished by a rash that may appear on the scalp, face, or neck, but it does not affect the internal organs. Normally, only about 10% of people who get this develop systemic lupus erythematosus. However, there is no way to predict or stop the disease's progression.

### ERYTHEMATOSUS DRUG-INDUCED

This type of Lupus develops as a result of a reaction to certain prescription drugs, and its symptoms are similar to systemic lupus erythematosus. This type of Lupus is linked to the use of hydralazine and procainamide, but nearly 400 other medications have been linked to it. This type of Lupus resolves after the patient discontinues the triggering medications.

### NEONATAL LUPUS

This uncommon form of Lupus develops when a mother passes autoantibodies to her fetus. Skin rashes, as well as other blood and heart complications, can occur in a newborn or unborn fetus. The rashes usually go away or fade within the first six months of a child's life.

### LUPUS ERYTHEMATOSUS SYSTEMIC

It is the most common and severe form of systemic Lupus, and it can affect any part of the body or organ. Some people with SLE may only have inflammation and other joint and skin symptoms, whereas others may have inflammation in joints, skin, or any other body organ. This type of Lupus is distinguished by flare-ups as well as periods of remission.

## WHO IS SUSCEPTIBLE TO LUPUS?

According to the Lupus Foundation of America, 1.5 to 2 million people in the United States have Lupus of some kind. Lupus affects 40 people out of every 100,000 people in Northern Europe. Lupus affects 200 African-Americans out of every 100,000. Although both males and females can be affected by Lupus, females are nine times more likely to develop this autoimmune disease. African American women have a higher mortality rate and a more severe form of this disorder. It primarily affects people aged 15 to 45. Other risk factors include some prescription medications, exposure to sunlight, and chemicals.

The true cause of this disease, like many other autoimmune diseases, is unknown; however, many healthcare professionals believe it is caused by genetic and environmental factors. Many doctors believe that because Lupus runs in families, people inherit a genetic predisposition to the disease from their parents. People who inherit a genetic predisposition to this disease are thought to develop it only when they are exposed to certain environmental triggers. The increased risk of Lupus in females suggests that certain hormones may play a role in the development of this disease.

Some Environmental Triggering Factors

- Smoking Excessive stress
- Being subjected to UV light
- Some medications in the sulpha and penicillin groups
- Having viral infections such as parvovirus, hepatitis C, and so on.

Lupus Signs and Symptoms

People with lupus will experience symptoms during flare-ups. In between flare-ups, people with lupus will have none or only a few symptoms.

Lupus manifests itself in a variety of ways, including:

- Arthritis
- Stress or cold can cause purple or pale toes or fingers.
- Unusual hair loss
- When taking deep breaths, I experience chest pain.
- Headaches
- Fever
- Sun sensitivity
- Ulcers in the mouth
- Rashes on the skin caused by bleeding beneath the skin
- Lymph nodes or glands that are swollen
- Swelling in the legs or around the eyes
- Muscle or joint swollenness or pain
- Loss of appetite and weight loss
- Fatigue

## *Lupus Complications*

Because Lupus is an autoinflammatory disease, inflammation caused by Lupus can affect various parts of the body.

### HEART

Lupus can inflame arteries, heart membranes, and heart muscles. Because of this inflammation, the risk of having a heart attack and developing heart disease may increase significantly.

### LUNGS

Lupus increases the likelihood of developing inflammation in the lining of the chest cavity. The resulting inflammation can make breathing more difficult. People who have Lupus are more prone to pneumonia.

### KIDNEYS

Lupus can cause serious kidney damage. Kidney failure is one of the leading causes of death in lupus patients. Among the obvious kidney problems are chest pain, vomiting, nausea, generalized itching, and leg edema.

### THE BLOOD AND THE BLOOD VESSELS

People with Lupus are more likely to develop blood problems such as anemia, blood clotting, and excessive bleeding. This disorder may cause blood vessels to become inflamed.

### THE CENTRAL NERVOUS SYSTEM AND THE BRAIN

People who have Lupus may develop brain and CNS issues. Behavioral changes, dizziness, light headaches, hallucinations, strokes, or seizures are all possible symptoms. Some people with lupus experience memory loss and difficulty expressing themselves to others.

### FACTORS OF RISK

Lupus can be caused by a variety of factors. As previously stated, these could be environmental, genetic, hormonal, or any combination of these. Let us be a little more specific:

### HISTORY OF THE FAMILY

Anyone with a first or second-degree relative who has lupus is at a higher risk of developing the disease. Scientists have discovered specific genes that may play a role in the development of lupus. Simply put, there hasn't been enough evidence to prove that they are the cause of the disease.

In some studies of identical twins, one twin may develop lupus while the other does not, even though they grew up together and were exposed to the same environmental factors. If one twin has lupus, the other has a 25% chance of developing the disease as well. This condition is more genetically imposed on identical twins.

Lupus can occur in people who have no family history of the disease, but there may be other autoimmune diseases in the family. Idiopathic thrombocytopenic purpura, hemolytic anemia, and thyroiditis are a few examples.

Changes to the X-chromosomes, according to some researchers, may increase the risk.

### RACE

Lupus can affect people of any ethnicity, but it is about three times more common in African-Americans than in Caucasians. It is also more common in women of Native American, Asian, and Hispanic descent.

### HORMONES

These are chemicals that the body produces. They aid in the regulation and control of specific organs or cells.

This hormonal activity could explain the following risk factors:

### AGE

The diagnosis and symptoms typically occur between the ages of 15 and 45, i.e., during a woman's childbearing years. However, approximately 20% of all cases occur after a woman reaches the age of 50.

Scientists have investigated a link between lupus and estrogen because nine out of ten lupus diagnoses are female. Women and men both produce estrogen, but women produce a greater amount.

In one study published in 2016, researchers discovered that estrogen can affect the immune activity and cause the development of lupus antibodies in women who are predisposed to the disease.

This could explain why women are more likely to be affected by autoimmune diseases than men. In 2010, researchers published a study that found women with lupus experienced more fatigue and pain during menstruation. This could imply that symptoms will worsen during this time.

There simply isn't enough evidence to conclude that estrogen causes lupus. If there is a true link, an estrogen-based treatment may be able to control how severe lupus becomes. Much more research is required before doctors can recommend it as a treatment.

### GUT MICROBIOTA

Recently, researchers have been looking at gut microbiota as one factor in the development of lupus. According to the researchers, specific changes in gut microbiota occurred in both mice and lupus patients. More research is needed in this area.

### Lupus Diagnosis

Lupus is difficult to diagnose because its symptoms overlap with those of many other diseases and conditions. There is no single test that can determine whether or not you have Lupus. In any case, if you have Lupus symptoms, contact your doctor or physician right away. Your doctor will determine whether or not you have Lupus.

### URINE AND BLOOD TESTS

Your physician will order an antinuclear antibody test. This test determines whether or not a person's immune system produces autoantibodies for Lupus. Surprisingly, the majority of people's ANA tests are usually positive. A positive ANA (antinuclear antibody) test, on the other hand, does not rule out Lupus. A small percentage of healthy women who do not have Lupus have a positive ANA test.

### MEDICAL HISTORY

Explain to your doctor your symptoms and signs. Your doctor can determine whether you have Lupus by reviewing your medical history.

Complete a physical examination

A thorough physical examination can assist a doctor in diagnosing this disease.

Lupus or other Autoimmune Diseases in the Family

Inform your doctor if you have a family history of Lupus or any other autoimmune disease. That could help your doctor make a more accurate diagnosis.

### KIDNEY OR SKIN BIOPSY

A kidney or skin biopsy can be used to help diagnose this disorder.

## Conventional Therapies

There is currently no cure for Lupus. As a result, the treatment goal is to reduce inflammation, alleviate symptoms, reduce the risk of organ damage, reduce flares, and treat symptoms as they appear.

Drug classes commonly used to treat Lupus include:

- Immunosuppressants
- NSAIDs, corticosteroids
- BLyS-specific inhibitors
- antimalarial medications
- anti-inflammatory diets

## Causes

We know Lupus is an autoimmune disease, but no specific cause has been identified.

Lupus is caused by our immune systems attacking healthy body tissues. Lupus is most likely the result of a combination of your environment and genetics.

If a person has an inherited predisposition to Lupus, they may develop the disease if they come into contact with something in their environment that triggers Lupus.

Our immune systems will defend our bodies and combat antigens such as germs, bacteria, and viruses. This occurs because it produces antibodies, which are proteins.

When you have an autoimmune disease, such as lupus, your immune system is unable to distinguish between healthy tissue, antigens, and unwanted substances. As a result, our immune system will direct antibodies to attack antigens as well as healthy tissues. This may result in tissue damage, pain, and swelling.

The most common type of autoantibody that develops in Lupus patients is an antinuclear antibody. This ANA binds to the nucleus of the cell. All of these autoantibodies circulate throughout the blood, but some cells have thin walls that allow autoantibodies to pass through.

These autoantibodies have the potential to attack the body's DNA in the nucleus of cells. That is why Lupus will affect some organs but not others.

Why Does the Immune System Fail?

Some genetic factors contribute to the development of SLE. Some genes in the body can aid in the proper functioning of the immune system. These changes may impair the ability of people with SLE's immune systems to function properly.

One theory relates to cell death. It is a natural process that occurs when the body renews its cells. Some scientists believe that genetic factors contribute to the body's inability to eliminate dead cells. Dead cells that remain in the body may release substances that cause the immune system to malfunction.

Can Children Be Put in Danger?

Lupus is extremely rare in children under the age of 15 if their birth mother did not have it. They may have lupus-related skin, liver, or heart problems if their birth mother had it.

Infants with neonatal lupus may be more likely to develop another autoimmune disease later in life.

## COMPLICATIONS OF AUTOIMMUNE DISEASES

*Cancer*

Cancer can start anywhere in the body. It begins when the cells multiply rapidly and take up the space normally occupied by normal cells. As a result, the body is unable to function normally.

That several people will cope well with cancer. More people are living longer lives as a result of cancer treatment than ever before.

We'll define cancer and discuss its causes here. Cancer is a collection of tumors, not a single disease. It is not just about one disorder. Cancer can start in the breast, the lungs, the colon, or the blood. Cancers are similar in some ways, but differ in how they develop and spread.

*How does cancer resemble each other?*

Our cells do have some functions in our bodies. Regular cells break in a predictable pattern. When they are stretched or injured, they die, and new cells form. Cancer develops when cells begin to develop out of balance. Cancer cells begin to grow and form new cells. The snare normal ones. This causes complications in the area of the body where cancer begins.

Cancerous cells frequently spread to other parts of the body. Lung cancer cells, for example, may migrate to and expand in the bones. As cancer cells spread, this is referred to as metastasis (meh-TASuh-sis). If lung cancer spreads to the bones, it is classified as a tumor of the lungs. The cancer cells, which are mostly found in bones, appear to be similar to those found in the lungs. If cancer began in the bones, it is referred to as bone cancer.

Some tumors are simple to form and spread. The other will gradually expand. They frequently respond to care in a variety of ways. Some cancers respond best to surgery, while others respond well to chemotherapy. Typically, two or three procedures are used to achieve the best results.

The specialist may want to know what type of cancer it is. Cancer patients require care that is tailored to their specific cancer type.

Many tumors form a lump known as a growing tumor. However, lumps aren't always cancer. Medical personnel is removing a piece of the swelling to look for cancer. Noncancerous bumps or lumps are referred to as benign. Malignant lumps are those that cause cancer.

Tumors of this type, such as leukemia (blood cancer), do not form. They develop in blood cells or other cells in the body.

"When you're told you're going to die from cancer, you're filled with dread. It is nearly impossible to care for anything other than the illness at first. This is the first thing you think or talk about every morning. I want cancer patients to believe that their situation is improving. Thinking about cancer allows you to cope with all of the different emotions you are experiencing. Remember that being upset is normal. " -Delores survivor of cancer

What causes cancer to develop?

Cancer can be caused by accumulated gene damage.

Such changes could be the result of chance or exposure to the cancer-causing substance.

Carcinogens are cancer-causing compounds. Carcinogens, such as some cigarette smoke compounds, can be chemical elements. Cancer can also be caused by bacteria, the environment, or a genetic mutation.

We can divide cancer risk factors into roughly the following groups:

1. Lifestyle-related factors
2. The environment
3. Bacteria and viruses
1. Lifestyle factors include:

- Alcohol
- Tobacco
- Several food-related factors, such as polyaromatic hydrocarbons and nitrites produced by the barbecue.

2. Some cancer-causing factors associated with one's living environment and place of employment include:

- Pitch and tar
- UV radiations
- Polynuclear hydrocarbons (e.g., benzopyrene) and asbestos fibers

- Certain metal compounds
- Certain toxic plastic chemicals (e.g., vinyl chloride)

3. Bacteria and viruses can cause cancer:

- Helicobacter pylori (the causative agent of gastritis)
- HCV, HBV (hepatitis virus causing hepatitis)
- HPV (human papillomavirus, papillomavirus that causes changes in cells, such as cervical cells)
- Epstein-Barr virus (herpes virus that causes lymphoid gland inflammation)

## Diabetes mellitus

Diabetes is a metabolic disorder characterized by elevated blood sugar levels. Insulin is a hormone that transports glucose from the blood into cells for energy absorption or utilization. Diabetes indicates that the body either does not produce enough insulin or does not use the insulin it does produce efficiently.

Untreated high diabetes blood sugar will harm your skin, nerves, kidneys, and other organs.

## Diseases and Dr. Sebi

What Is the Cause of Disease and How Do I Get Rid of It?

"Disease is an illness affecting humans, animals, or plants, often caused by infection," according to Oxford learners dictionaries, whereas Dr. Sebi defines disease as "the compromising of the mucous membrane."

When I say the mucous membrane is compromised, I mean that it has been broken. So, the location of the broken or compromised mucous membrane determines the illness that will manifest.

He goes on to say that there is only one disease, which is mucus (inflammation). " Take it or leave it, there is only one disease, and mucus is the source of all diseases.

The table below shows where the mucous membrane is compromised and the illnesses that result:

| S/No. | Point of Membrane Compromised | Sickness |
|---|---|---|
| I. | Lungs | Pneumonia, cystic fibrosis, (COPD) chronic obstructive pulmonary disease |
| Ii. | Bronchial Tubes | Bronchitis |
| III. | Trachea | Hemopytsis, wheezing and Stridor |
| Iv. | Reproductive Organ | Fibroid or low sperm counts, infertility, endometriosis and so on. |

| V. | Pancreatic Duct | Diabetes |
|---|---|---|
| Vi. | Eye Retina | Blindness or Blur Sight |
| Vii. | Kidney | Kidney stone, acute kidney injury and so on |
| Viii. | Brain | Parkinson, paranoia, insomnia and so on. |
| IX. | Joint | Arthritis |
| X | Heart | Heart Failure, high/lo blood pressure etc. |

This is why Dr. Sebi opposes cleansing only one part of the body, the colon, and instead believes in cleansing the entire body system. Because the entire body is interconnected, the only way to eliminate the root cause of hypertension, according to late Dr. Sebi, is through intracellular cleansing (cleansing/detoxification) of the whole cells. Cleaning one cell without cleaning the others is the same as not cleaning because the unclean cells will infect the clean cells.

So, undergoing an intracellular cleansing means that you are resetting your entire cells from the colon to the lymph glands, liver, gallbladder, kidney, and skin back to their original state (alkaline environment) where no disease can withstand and revitalizing the body system to recover from the energy that it has lost due to the presence of the disease.

What Are The Foundations For Self-Healing From ADs?

The following rules must be followed to treat autoimmune diseases naturally:

1. Adhere to Dr. Sebi's nutritional guidelines religiously.
2. Drink at least one gallon of spring water per day.
3. Use only a small amount of sea salt and avoid table salt entirely.
4. Avoid eating too much grain, including alkaline grain.
5. Check to see if you have a kidney or thyroid disorder.

## HEALING FROM AN AUTOIMMUNE DISEASE WITH DR. SEBI'S TREATMENTS

According to Dr. Sebi, if the body is not nourished with alkaline foods and herbs, it can experience six stages of over-acidity:

1. Perceptiveness - You'll know you're in this stage if you start having low energy, acne, or a bad odor.
2. Irritation - The following one is where you begin to experience bowel diseases such as IBS, constipation, and diarrhea.
3. Mucus Production - This is the point at which your body can no longer tolerate living in an extra-acidic environment and begins producing mucus to try to protect itself.

4. Irritation - When mucus begins to accumulate, your body responds by initiating the inflammatory process. This could lead to you developing Arthritis or Fibromyalgia.

5. Indulgences - Atherosclerosis, also known as "artery hardening," is the most dangerous complication at this stage. When mucus begins to deposit in them, it is referred to as 'plaques.' These plaques can narrow or block the arteries over time, causing unpredictable problems such as strokes.

6. Degeneration - In the final stage, mucus begins to accumulate in the brain, bones, and nerves. If this occurs, dangerous diseases such as cancer, Multiple Sclerosis, or osteoporosis may develop.

Dr. Sebi's official method for treating autoimmune diseases consists of three major steps. Please keep in mind that any of these components cannot be skipped for your healing journey to be successful.

The three steps I'm referring to are as follows:

1. Decontamination - During the first stage, your body must be cleansed on an intracellular level through detoxification to purify each cell and remove excess mucus

2. Rejuvenating - After cleansing, you should nourish your body, regenerate your cells, and strengthen your immune system.

3. Maintaining the Immune System's Health - You can keep your mind sharp and your immune system strong by following Dr. Sebi's nutrition guide and adopting healthy lifestyle habits every day.

*First Stage: Cleansing*

## HOW DO YOU MAKE CLEANSING HERBS?

The way you prepare your cleansing herbs will be heavily influenced by the form in which you purchased them. Cleansing herbs are easier to prepare in powder form because you can easily make herbal teas with them in the specified or recommended dosage. However, for other forms of herbs, particularly roots or leaves, a ratio of 1 teaspoon to 1 cup (8 oz) of spring water is preferable.

However, I recommend preparing herbs in batches of mixtures for easier batch preparation and storage. That would imply combining them based on function and benefit. Again, this will be determined by your current state of health and the minerals that are most important to you. You can make a batch of similar herbs with similar functions. Overall, try not to combine more than two or three herbs. Remember, these herbs are electric, and we should do everything we can to preserve their organic carbon, hydrogen, and oxygen nature. Once again, if you More than that, and you may not get accurate concentrations per ml of water, so try to keep it to three or two.

You can use the following combination for a better understanding:

- Combine colon and gallbladder cleansing herbs.
- Combine liver and kidney cleansing herbs.
- Combine herbs for respiratory and mucus cleansing.
- Combine lymphatic and heavy-metal cleansing herbs in a tea.

Because these herbs cleanse the entire body (not just the colon), including the skin, eyes, colon, liver, lymphatic system, and gallbladder, you can choose how to combine them. Also, when making larger batches of these herbs for storage, try not to make batches that will last longer than 7 to 14 days.

Cleansing Packages can be pre-purchased.

Please adhere to the recommended dosage or instructions for that cleansing package.

### Green Leafy Herbs

- Boil fresh green leafy herbs in spring water for 5 to 7 minutes on low heat.
- Boil dried leafy herbs for 10 to 15 minutes on low heat.

Herbs, dried ground (or powder)

Mix dried ground or powdered leaves or roots in the herb's recommended ratios. Powder herbs are the simplest to combine in dosage proportions, so simply follow the package directions.

### For Dried Root Herb Chunks

If you bought chunks of roots or stems, you can prepare them as follows:

- Cut or break up chunks - Place in a pot of boiling water for 15 minutes
- Allow cooling before serving.
- Alternatively, make larger batches and store them in jars in the refrigerator.

Herbs can be purchased in bulk.

If you bought your herbs in bulk and are making tea, find out what the recommended dosage is for each herb. As a general rule, 1 teaspoon to 8 ounces of spring water should be used to make each herbal tea.

1 teaspoon Herb + 1 cup (8oz) Spring Water

For capsules

I recommend researching to determine the recommended dosage for each herbal capsule.

How To Use Cleansing Herbs That Have Been Prepared

If you are on medication, I recommend taking the herbs one hour before taking your meds, as Dr. Sebi suggested. Your colon cleansing herbs should not be taken for more than 30 days because your body may become dependent on them, and you should begin reducing the dose during the last 3 to 5 days, depending on how long you've been taking them.

Routine:

- Twice a day, in the morning and at night
- Day-to-day Consistency - Try to be consistent in terms of both timing and duration. To put it another way, try not to skew the duration. Make it a habit to consume the cleansing herb throughout the cleanse. For example, for a 14-day cleanse, the cleansing herbs can be taken twice daily, and they should be taken at the same time in the mornings and evenings.
- Gradual Weaning Off – Just like with medications, going cold turkey when it comes to herbal detox is not recommended. Wean off your herbs near the end of the cleanse by gradually reducing

the dosage and duration. The length of the wean will be determined by the length of the fast. For example, for a one-month fast, I usually begin weaning a week before the fast's end. I start weaning on day 11 or 12 of a 14-day fast. You can start the weaning process by reducing the dose from twice a day to once a day. Alternatively, divide the dosages in half for mornings and nights.

You must do this because you must signal your body to begin preparing to function independently without relying on herbs for cleansing.

## CAUSES OF CHRONIC KIDNEY DISEASE AND KIDNEY FAILURE

*Causes and Risk Factors*

Many of us are not aware that the cause of kidney disease doesn't necessarily have to occur in the kidneys themselves. Problems affecting our overall health and well-being can also induce damage to the kidneys. In the same way, common health problems can also impair the function of these organs. The most frequent causes of kidney disease are hypertension and diabetes.

High blood pressure, which affects 75 million people in the US or one in three adults, can damage blood vessels in the kidney and impair their function. In other words, damage to blood vessels in the kidneys due to hypertension doesn't allow them to remove wastes and extra fluid from your body. That leads to a vicious cycle as an accumulation of waste, and extra fluid increases blood pressure. Besides damaging filtering units in kidneys, high blood pressure can also reduce blood flow to these organs. As you're already aware, without a blood supply, organs cannot function properly.

About 30.3 million people, or 9.4% of the United States population, have diabetes, causing several complications. Just like hypertension, diabetes also damages small blood vessels in the kidneys. As a result, the body retains more salt and water than it should. Moreover, diabetes also damages the body's nerves, making it difficult for you to empty the bladder. The pressure from a full bladder can back up and damage or injure kidneys. Let's also not forget that if urine remains in the body for a long time, it can lead to an infection from the fast growth of bacteria and high blood sugar levels. Estimates show that 30% of patients with type 1 diabetes and 10% to 40% of people with type 2 diabetes will eventually experience kidney failure.

Besides diabetes and hypertension, other causes of kidney disease include:

- Infection
- Renal artery stenosis
- Heavy metal poisoning
- Lupus
- Some drugs
- Prolonged obstruction of the urinary tract from conditions such as kidney stones, enlarged prostate, some cancers

# SYMPTOMS OF CKD

One way to help a person know if he or she is suffering from chronic kidney disease is to be informed about its signs and symptoms.

When these signs and symptoms show, immediately seek the assistance of medical experts to avoid complications.

The common signs of chronic kidney disease are:

- Nausea and Vomiting. When you experience nausea, you sense discomfort in your upper stomach. You get a sensation of uneasiness and an urge to vomit involuntarily. Most of the time, a person vomits after experiencing nausea.
- Loss of Appetite. Changes in your eating habits may be a sign that you are already suffering from chronic kidney disorder. When you begin to notice that you are eating less than usual or are not feeling any urge or motivation to eat at all for no apparent reason, it is time that you consult your doctor. Not only is it a sign of chronic kidney disease, but loss of appetite may also result in weight loss and malnutrition.
- Changes in urination. Whether you are urinating more or less than usual or are experiencing changes in your urine's color, you should seek medical assistance. We know for a fact that the kidneys are the ones responsible for the production of urine. If there are changes in urination, this means that there are changes in the functioning of the kidney as well. It may be a sign of improvement for some but can be very risky for many. You know that you are experiencing changes in urination when you frequently need to wake up in the middle of the night just to urinate, your urine has a bubble or is foamy, when it contains blood, dark-colored. You urinate less frequently and in smaller amounts, or whenever you feel difficulty or pressure when urinating.
- Swelling. Swelling may occur whenever you are injured or when you accidentally bumped into something hard. However, if you experience swelling without any external cause, then this may be a sign that your kidneys are beginning to fail. Swelling occurs because the kidneys are no longer able to remove the extra fluids in your body. Swelling may occur in the ankles, legs, feet, hands, or face.
- Fatigue. The kidneys produce hormones responsible for keeping us energetic every day. When they fail, our bodies also fail to receive and carry oxygen, making our brains and muscles tire quickly.
- Itching or Skin Rash. One of the kidneys' main functions is to filter the blood and remove the bloodstream wastes when the kidneys fail to function properly; these wastes build-up, causing itching and skin rash.
- Shortness of Breath. When the kidneys fail to remove extra fluid in our body, they can stay in the lungs and build up in there. Kidney can also trigger the development of anemia. When anemia is complicated, your body will starve for oxygen. Thus, one experiences shortness of breath.
- Trouble concentrating and dizziness. As mentioned earlier, different parts of the body fail to receive and carry oxygen due to kidney failure. One of these is the brain. If the brain fails to get enough oxygen, you may experience dizziness, memory problems, and inability to focus properly.

Other minor signs may be:

- Weight loss
- Blood in urine
- Insomnia
- Muscle cramps
- Erectile dysfunction in men

Now that you know the signs and symptoms of chronic kidney disease, it is easier for you to detect whether you are suffering from it or not. However, knowing the signs and symptoms is not enough.

## CORRELATION WITH OTHER DISEASES

According to experts, the renal disease requires early diagnosis and targeted treatment to prevent or delay both a condition of acute or chronic renal failure and the appearance of cardiovascular complications to which it is often associated.

Hypertension and diabetes, not adequately controlled by drug therapy, prostatic hypertrophy, kidney stones, or bulky tumors, can promote onset. They reduce the normal flow of urine and increase the kidneys' pressure and limit functionality.

Or the kidney damage can be determined by inflammatory processes (pyelonephritis, glomerulonephritis) or by the formation of cysts inside the kidneys (polycystic kidney disease) or by the chronic use of some drugs, alcohol, and drugs consumed in excess.

A fundamental role in alleviating the already compromised kidneys' work is the diet, the first prevention. It must be studied with an expert nutritionist or a nephrologist to maintain or reach an ideal weight on the one hand and on the other to reduce the intake of sodium (salt), and the consequent control of blood pressure, and other substances (minerals), without creating malnutrition or nutritional deficiencies. Particular attention should also be paid to cholesterol, triglycerides, and blood sugar levels.

Understanding what causes kidney failure goes a long way to deciding just what kind of treatment you should focus on. The most important factor that you should focus on is, of course, your diet. But as you focus on your diet, make sure that you are following your doctor's instructions in the event of other complications. Let us look at a few of the common causes of kidney diseases.

### Diabetes

Diabetes causes damages to the different organs in our bodies, including:

- Heart
- Kidneys
- Eyes
- Nerves
- Blood vessels

*High Blood Pressure*

Thus, a person must watch over his diet and the activities he engages in to avoid hypertension. Although it is a common health problem, it still poses serious risks and complications.

The risk factors for hypertension include age, obesity, family history, smoking, lack of exercise, stress, excessive alcohol consumption, high fat diet, and sodium intake.

An important thing to remember here is that high blood pressure can be both a cause and CKD symptom, similar to diabetes.

So, what exactly is blood pressure? People often throw the term around, but they cannot pinpoint what happens when the blood pressure increases.

*Malformations*

Even when you are still in your mother's womb, risks of developing chronic kidney disease are already present. Mothers should be extra cautious when pregnant because preventing urine outflow may affect the baby's organs.

*Lupus*

Systemic lupus erythematous causes the body's immune system to attack the kidney even if it is not a foreign tissue. It may take a long time before a person recovers from lupus because it eventually goes back after some time, but it is possible through proper treatments.

*Obstructions*

Obstructions or blockages such as tumors, kidney stones, or enlarged prostate gland can trigger chronic kidney disease development.

The causes mentioned above are just the most common of the many causes of chronic kidney disease. There are cases when CKD is caused not only by a single factor. Sometimes, a combination of these factors causes the development of chronic kidney disease.

Nonetheless, a patient needs to know the cause of their condition to be prescribed with the proper treatments and medications.

Kidneys may be small, but they do have important functions in the body. These bean-shaped organs work hard, but they may experience injuries and other problems that prevent them from functioning properly. But the question is, what causes kidney disease and how to detect it?

## DR. SEBI'S TREATMENTS FOR KIDNEYS HEALTH

*How did dr. Sebi address kidney diseases?*

Dr. Sebi said, "Detoxification is at the heart of getting rid of kidney problems associated with mucus out of the body; there are no other ways that will bring the required result." Therefore, fasting is an essential factor that can help detoxify the body, especially the kidney. Fasting helps your body, including the blood, kidney, and liver, to experience cleansing and detoxification. To achieve a cure for kidney problems, you have to be willing to make a sacrifice like the one you are about to undergo.

Detoxifying your body could end your kidney problems, depending on how serious you engage in the methods, since they are not easy to eliminate.

## Treatment and Passing of Kidney Stones

The treatment of kidney stones requires the intake of alkaline herbs beneficial for consumption as food and medicinal herbs. That means you have to consider both methods to be able to fight kidney abnormalities and problems.

The diet, which comprises vegetables, fruits, and grains, contains high amounts of magnesium and calcium because a reduced amount of these minerals could result in kidney stones problems.

Herbs can are very effective for fighting stones, and some of them are also very common

The herbs perform their functions by relieving edema in the ureter mucosa, decreasing spasms that occur due to kidney stones' irritation, and improving urine flow.

Examples of these herbs are:

1.  Saw Palmetto Fruit

Saw palmetto fruit contains many ethyl esters of fatty acids, enzymes, tannins, resins, terpenoids, and sitosterols.

It is a reliable plant used for the treatment of Benign Prostate Hyperplasia (BPH). The herb contains a tonic that helps the urinary tract, and it is used for both male and female sufferers.

This fruit contains spasmolytic effects, making it easy to remove stones, and it also benefits patients with dysuria and tenesmus. This herb reduces the bladder's pressure and has a sedative effect on an irritated detrusor, which assists sufferers with bladder and prostate abnormalities.

2.  Dandelion Leaf

This plant leaf is very effective in the detoxification of the liver and kidney. The leaf is a strong diuretic, and it is compared to furosemide in animal studies. It has also been carried out in humans, and it was discovered that the effects are similar. Animal studies have shown that dandelion leaf is important in removing kidney stones via the direct passage.

Dandelion is one of the major sources of potassium, with about 4.25% potassium compared to other drugs, containing a lesser amount. It can be used as a diet and medication because of its ability to improve its urinary and biliary system.

3.  Lobelia Flower, Seed, and Leaf

Lobelia contains powerful relaxant and antispasmodic effects that assist the urinary stones to pass through the ureters easily. This plant is regarded as acetylcholine antagonists though other mechanisms may speak for its broncho and ureter-relaxing effects.

4.  Goldenrod Leaf or Flower

This herb is used as a strong urinary stimulant, improving diuresis and reducing albuminuria in the kidney.

It is also very important for nephritis treatment and helps stabilize the body immediately after the kidney has discharged the stones. That means it should be used immediately after the kidney stone has been ejected.

The presence of flavonoids in the plant helps repair the kidney, blood vessels, and connective tissues surrounding the kidney.

5. Horsetail Leaf

Horsetail leaf effectively repairs connective tissues surrounding the kidney and the lungs due to a silica component.

Horsetail also helps in diuresis, and it is a general metabolic stimulant that increases connective tissue resistance. It is important in both acute and chronic removal of kidney stones.

6. Khella Seed

Khella plant, especially the seed, contains khellin and visnadin as their active components, making it useful by acting as a mild calcium channel blocker in the ureters' dilation.

Visnadin contains some smooth-muscle relaxing components which is associated with the non-standard calcium-channel activity.

The active components present in Khella seed are excellently absorbed and have reduced toxicity as evidenced by the almost total lack of side effects with long-term use in treating an individual with asthma.

7. Corn Silk

Corn silk is a very important herb as it is used to increase the easy flow of urine. It contains a demulcent property that helps reduce irritation from stones and facilitate its easy removal.

This plant should be collected fresh, especially when it is still very green, to prevent the consumption of a low-quality herb.

8. Madder Root

Madder root is significant and used by patients with kidney problems because it has a spasmolytic effect on the ureters and enables the free passage of stones. This plant was studied, and it has been proved to contain calcium-channel antagonizing effects, which might contribute to relaxing the muscles.

This plant is also used to prevent calcium and phosphate oxalate salts from forming kidney stones in the body.

9. Gravel Root

This plant is used for the treatment of the urinary tract.

Gravel root can dissolve concretions. It is used for the treatment of urethritis, cystitis, irritable bladder, and fluid retention.

10. Horse Chestnut Fruit

This plant is used to treat various health conditions because of anti-edema properties known as escin. Escin reduces the small pore number and diameter in capillary endothelium, thereby decreasing fluid seepage into the tissues (Longiave D. et al. 1978).

The presence of calculi in the ureter is easily removed with the use of this plant. The plant has anti-edema properties that help in the production of enlargement of the internal diameter of the ureter, thereby helping the stones to migrate easily even in resistant cases.

11. Couch Grass

This plant is a saponin and mannitol-containing diuretic that contain some silica. This herb helps in the repair of irritated mucous walls and has been used to treat prostatic adenoma.

This plant helps in the easy removal of stones and helps repair and prevent kidney stones' recurrence.

12. Hydrangea Root

This plant is important and useful for the easy removal of stones. It is also helpful for sufferers who have urinary tract infections and prostate enlargement.

Foods to Limit to Safeguard Kidney Function

We have already seen a lot of the food that you should avoid. For that reason, I am going to include a few more to the list, explain why they should be avoided, and then I am going to show you some incredible spice blends and seasonings that you can use on your food.

Let's start with some foods that you should avoid.

## Whole-Wheat Bread

Normally, whole-wheat bread is considered a healthy option. But for people with kidney diseases, that is not the case. The reason for this is that the more whole-wheat and bran in bread, the more potassium and phosphorus content you are likely to find in them.

A 30 gram (or 1 ounce) serving of whole-wheat bread could contain around 68 mg of potassium and 57 mg of phosphorus, and if you eat plenty of it, that would potentially be too much for your kidneys.

## Brown Rice

The case for avoiding brown rice is similar to the one made to avoid whole-wheat bread; it contains too much potassium and phosphorus for your body to handle. A single cup of brown rice contains about 154 mg of potassium and around 150 mg of phosphorus. Compare that to a cup of white rice, and the difference is remarkable; you will find just 54 mg of potassium and around 68 mg of phosphorus in the white rice. That's less than half the amount that brown rice has!

If you feel that you do not want to include white rice into the diet, try alternatives to brown rice such as couscous, bulgur, buckwheat, and pearled barley. They are not only nutritious but delicious as well.

## *Dairy*

Milk is often recommended for strong bones and muscles. But for those with kidney diseases, having milk increases the potassium and phosphorus content in the blood. It might be important for people to consume milk in many cases since it aids them with other medical conditions. If you require milk in your diet, ensure that you communicate your medical history, issues, current diet, and other vital information to your doctor. By doing so, you will get proper recommendations on how you can include milk in your diet.

When you visit your doctor, make sure that you are completely honest about your medical history, habits, and diet. Don't try to hide the fact that you occasionally sneak in a cup of that good, sweet, chilled soda pop in the middle of the night. Don't be embarrassed to admit something if it concerns your kidneys or your health. Your doctors are not there to judge you. Trust me; there is nothing you can say that they haven't seen or heard before. And in some cases, what they might have experienced could be quite shocking or surprising to you.

# DR. SEBI ANXIETY SOLUTION

## RISKS FACTORS FOR ANXIETY

### Neuroanatomy

The neural structures involved in the functioning of anxiety include Amygdala (which is the center for emotions such as anxiety and fear and stimulates the Sympathetic nervous system), Hippocampus (which is the center for emotional memory). People experiencing high levels of anxiety have been seen to have highly stimulated Amygdala and hippocampus. Many researches regarding teenagers who were recorded to be more apprehensive, cautious, and fearful in their childhood have shown that their nucleus accumbens are much more sensitive than other people, especially when deciding about a reward gaining situation. This automatically concludes a relationship between the structures that control reward and fear responses in anxiety suffering people.

### Genetics

A family history of anxiety and genetic material is a huge risk factor contributing to anxiety. It renders a person vulnerable to anxiety disorders. Still, this anxiety disorder comes into action when triggered by specific stimuli, usually external and environmental. This genetic factor has contributed to 3% of anxiety disorders, and in 28% of the cases suffering from generalized anxiety disorder. No complete single gene has been found to cause anxiety by itself.

Several parts of certain genes have been proven to contribute to anxiety, such as:

- PLXNA2
- CRH
- BDNF
- COMT
- SERT.

The mode of action for these genes to cause anxiety is their action on the neurotransmitters, e.g., epinephrine and serotonin, and some stress hormones such as cortisol, which have been seen in anxiety disorders.

### Medical conditions

There are a huge number of medical conditions that can result in anxiety. Some of these medical conditions include breathing problems such as Asthma and COPD and the breathing problems experienced when on a death bed. Abdominal pain and chest causing medical conditions can also cause anxiety. Sometimes, these conditions are usually somatic representations of anxiety, the same as for sexual disorders. In teenagers, any conditions that affect the appearance, such as skin and face conditions, trigger social anxiety. In children, one of the main causes of social anxiety is a developmental disability. Similarly, chronic and fatal diseases, such as cancer, can also cause severe anxiety. Even so, many organic medical conditions cause symptoms mimicking anxiety.

Some of these medical conditions include:

- Endocrine diseases, such as hypo or hyperthyroidism
- Metabolic syndromes, e.g., diabetes, deficiency conditions such as deficiency of vitamins B2, B12, D, etc.
- Gastric diseases, such as celiac, gluten sensitivity, bowel diseases, etc.
- Heart conditions and blood diseases, like anemia
- Cerebral accidents, like strokes and tumors etc.
- Degenerative diseases of the brain, like Parkinson's, Multiple Sclerosis, Alzheimer's, dementia, Huntington's Chorea, and many more.

## Substance-induced

There are many drugs that their uses can precipitate or increase the levels of already existing anxiety. It does not matter whether the drug is being used for intoxication or the person is a heavy user or going through withdrawal of the drug. Some of these drugs include Tobacco, Cannabis, sedatives (Benzodiazepines), alcohol, opioids such as pain killers that have been prescribed or illegal drugs like heroin, CNS stimulants like caffeine, amphetamines, and cocaine, hallucinogens like LSD, and inhaled drugs like Crack. The ironic part here is that some people use these drugs to self-medicate themselves for already existing anxiety. Still, these drugs treat anxiety for a short period, after which the person becomes tolerant to their effect, and his anxiety worsens.

## Psychological

Insufficient coping skills such as inflexibility, rigidity, inability to solve problems, denial, defense mechanisms, impulsive behavior, avoiding problems, instability, and escaping from threatening situations instead of focusing on solving them, are all related to causing or worsening already existing anxiety. Anxiety is also related to how a person has negative or pessimistic views about his future outcomes and how effectively they deal with the negativity in their life.

Some psychological dispositions like: catastrophizing about the future, over-generalizing everything, attempting to read minds, binocular tricks, reasoning about emotions, and mental filtering can cause anxiety.

The psychodynamic theory of psychology suggests that anxiety results from different unconscious conflicts between your fears and desires. These conflicts are between the three forces of our psyche called id, ego, and superego. These conflicts end in anxiety, and the ego employs defense mechanisms to overcome this anxiety. Some of these defense mechanisms are:

- Suppression
- Anticipation
- Repression
- Somatization

- Sublimation
- Repression
- Dissociation
- Etc.

For example: a child taught that anger is a negative emotion and never allowed to be angry will learn to repress his anger to avoid anxiety caused by disapproving parents on his anger. These types of conflicts causing anxiety can be managed with the help of psychodynamic therapy.

## Evolutionary psychology

From the perspective of evolutionary psychology, anxiety is good for us because it helps us remain cautious against all possible threats that we can face in our environment and help us devise ways to avoid that threat. That may be true to some extent. Still, the thing to remember is that a person who suffers from anxiety starts avoiding all environments and situations that may not be dangerous. This is why people suffering from anxiety don't usually die due to accidents, as they avoid every situation that can be potentially threatening or dangerous.

## Social

The social risk factors of anxiety range from trauma history, such as:

- Emotional or physical abuse in childhood or teenage
- Negative experiences in childhood
- Bad parenting
- Rejecting
- Hostile parents
- Harsh treatment
- High discipline
- No maternal warmth
- Anxious household environment
- Drug abuse
- Dysfunctional parents
- And neglect of children.

## Gender socialization

Some other factors based on context that have been seen to contribute to anxiety causation are Gender socialization and learning experiences. The learning mastery is the extent to which people think they control their own lives and instrumentality, which means factors like confidence about self-independence control the relationship between gender and anxiety.

## CONVENTIONAL TREATMENTS

Medication is one treatment option. Going for medication first may be right for who you are, but it is not the only option. Medication may be the best treatment; however, there are side effects with drugs.

Medication can also stop working. When medication stops working—what can you do? You have other drugs to try, but wouldn't it be nice if you could rely on other treatments available?

Keep in mind that you do have alternatives. When medication is right for you—use it. Treatment can involve both therapy and drugs. You may be on medication for the long-term or short-term. The choice is the psychiatrists, typically based on the severity of your anxiety disorder.

Medication takes time to be effective. After three months, you may see the actual results of the drug you have chosen to use. Medication does not completely cure anxiety disorders. Still, they are very helpful in treating and managing the symptoms of anxiety. A doctor or medical health professional should only give medication for anxiety, not by yourself. Some authentic psychologist with the license to practice can also prescribe medication. Medication can be used in two ways. It can be used as the sole treatment for anxiety or used after psychotherapy has already been applied. No improvements were observed with psychotherapy. But to achieve the best results and obtain a faster recovery, it is better to combine the use of psychotherapy and medication

The medication used for treating anxiety disorders is most commonly anti-depressants, anti-anxiety meds, and beta-blockers. These medicines only work if used regularly, and if their use is stopped, the anxiety symptoms will reemerge.

## Antidepressants

Antidepressants are the main meds used for treating depression, but they work just to treat anxiety disorders. Their working duration is several weeks, and they must be used regularly. Their side effects include nausea, headache, and insomnia. These side effects are not usually severe and are not a huge problem for users if the dose is adjusted so that you start from very light doses and then move on to increase quantity in small amounts over time.

## Anti-Anxiety Medications

The anti-anxiety medication helps in elevating the anxiety symptoms, and the panic attacks often experienced with them. The most commonly used anti-anxiety meds are the benzodiazepines. Benzodiazepines are the only meds used for the treatment of generalized anxiety disorder. Panic disorders and social phobia are also treated by using benzodiazepines, but Antidepressants best treat them.

## Beta-Blockers

Beta-blockers like atenolol and propranolol are very useful when treating the different anxiety symptoms, especially social anxiety disorder's physical symptoms. Doctors prescribe these medicines to overcome shaking, blushing, and trembling, and increasing heart rate when anxious.

Selecting the right kind of medicine for you, the right dose of that medicine, and the exact treatment method should be carefully adjusted to a person's unique needs and symptoms. They should be managed by an expert medical healthcare professional. It is only an expert who can tell you about each treatment plan's pros and cons and help you decide which one is best for you. Your doctor may have to try different methods and medicines with you before arriving at the right one.

You should make a point of discussing the following things with your doctor:

- Is the medication working for you or not, or to the extent it has improved your symptoms?
- The pros and cons of each type of medicines, especially the side effects
- Depending upon your medical history, which side effect can harm you the most
- The different changes you will be required to make in your lifestyle for your medication
- How much each medicine costs, and what are the other cheaper alternatives
- Other alternatives that you can explore regards to your anxiety such as vitamin intake, therapies, and supplements that may affect your meds

You should stop using medicines because some medicines cause serious side effects if their use is stopped suddenly. They should be discontinued slowly and gradually with the help of a doctor's advice.

## Selective Serotonin Reuptake Inhibitors

SSRIs or 'Selective Serotonin Reuptake Inhibitors relieve symptoms by blocking serotonin's absorption in your nerve cells. The drug works on the nerve cells in your brain. Serotonin affects your mood; therefore, blocking the uptake of serotonin enhances your mood. SSRIs typically prescribed include:

- Citalopram
- Fluoxetine
- Sertraline
- Escitalopram
- Paroxetine

This category of drugs offers fewer side effects than other medications such as tricyclic antidepressants. Common side effects of these drugs include sleepiness, insomnia, weight gain, and sexual dysfunction.

## Tricyclic Antidepressants and Benzodiazepines

This classification of medicines replaced benzodiazepines due to concerns of long-term use by patients. Benzodiazepines help induce relaxation, reduce muscular tension, and alleviate many symptoms of anxiety. However, long-term use of Benzodiazepines leads to dependence and tolerance of the drug. They become ineffective.

Tricyclic antidepressants include:

- Imipramine
- Amitriptyline
- Nortriptyline
- Benzodiazepines are:
- Diazepam
- Alprazolam
- Lorazepam
- Clonazepam

Patients on tricyclic antidepressants may drop in blood pressure, urinary retention, constipation, blurry vision, or dry mouth.

*Serotonin-Norepinephrine Reuptake Inhibitors*

SNRIs like Duloxetine and Venlafaxine increase serotonin and norepinephrine by inhibiting their absorption in the brain cells. SNRIs can cause insomnia, stomachaches, headaches, increased blood pressure, or sexual dysfunction. Most doctors choose SSRIs or SNRIs before benzodiazepines or tricyclic antidepressants.

*Ketamine*

The recent clinical trials using Ketamine are favorable. Ketamine helps alleviate depression in a few hours, and some patients in minutes. The reaction time is faster than other medicines available. However, it is for depression—it will only relieve one symptom of your anxiety.

What You Should Know About Medications

If you take other medicines for other health conditions, anxiety meds may cause drug interactions. You should let your mental health provider know about any prescriptions, over-the-counter medications, vitamins, or supplements that you take.

Speak with your doctor or psychiatrist about medications they may want to take. If it will help you, what the side effects are, avoid certain things or drug interactions.

Pharmacists recommend you drink or eat before taking your pills and suggest a time to take them. These recommendations are to prevent side effects and to help your body absorb the substance correctly.

Before you decide to start medication for anxiety, discuss how long you may be on the meds with your doctor. Also, schedule a check-up to discuss how you feel about the medicine and if you need to extend the amount of time you will need to be on medication.

Due to dependency on drugs, you should carefully review the drug information and decide if it is right. You have other treatment options that may work better or work in conjunction with the meds to overcome your anxiety. If you find it necessary, obtain a second opinion. If you feel your doctor or psychiatrist is pushing medicine, speak with another mental health care worker.

## HOW ANXIETY IMPROVES WITH THE ALKALINE DIET

*Correct Nutrition can Help with Anxiety Disorder*

Based on research from the Mental Health Institute, anxiety disorders are more common than any other mental illness in America. That means that 18 percent of United States citizens suffer from anxiety symptoms. Depression and anxiety go together frequently, and about 50 percent of depression sufferers experience anxiety regularly in their lives. Some medications and therapies can reduce anxiety, but only 30 percent of people (or less) seek out professional help for their condition. But there are changes that you can make right at home to start helping your anxiety. Along with the techniques and mindset changes we've already discussed, like meditation and floating through the anxious thoughts, changing your diet can help you manage your nervousness and anxiety.

What is the Ideal Type of Diet for Lower Levels of Anxiety?

Most people know that eating healthy foods, drinking a lot of water throughout the day, and avoiding or limiting caffeine and alcohol is ideal for being healthy. However, there are other nutritional considerations you can make to help manage your anxiety. For example, complex carbs get metabolized slower by your body and keep your blood sugar maintained and level, promoting calmer moods and less anxiety. Eating foods based on fruit, vegetables, and whole grains, is better than eating processed, boxed foods and simple carbs like bread. The time of day that you eat matters as well, and you should never skip meals. Fasting too much can cause your blood sugar levels to drop and cause you to feel more anxious than usual.

Which Foods should you eat?

A lot of people don't realize that certain foods can lower levels of anxiety. You can start taking control of your levels of nervousness by being more conscious about what you eat.

Here are some examples of that:

FOODS WITH MAGNESIUM: In studies done on lab mice, nutritional diets that didn't have much magnesium, higher levels of anxiety were noticed. That means that foods with a lot of magnesium could help with general calm, such as Swiss chard, spinach, nuts, legumes, whole grains, and seeds.

PROBIOTIC FOOD SOURCES: A study done by the Psychiatric Research journal showed that there could be a link between lower anxiety levels and probiotic foods. Foods like sauerkraut, pickles, and kefir have been linked to lessened anxiety symptoms.

OMEGA-3 SOURCES: Omega-3 fatty acids might also help lower anxiety levels, based on a study done in 2011 on students in the medical field. This research utilized omega-3 supplements.

The government in China approved asparagus extract to be used for anti-anxiety purposes due to its beneficial properties. It also helps to eat foods like almonds and avocados, which are rich in vitamin B. Feel-good food sources like this result in dopamine and serotonin being released and are the easy, first step for managing your levels of anxiety at home.

Can Antioxidants help with your anxiety?

Low levels of antioxidants in the body are related to a higher state of anxiety. This means that including more antioxidant-rich foods in your daily diet can help you experience fewer symptoms and feel calmer, in general. A study done in the year 2010 looked at over 3,000 foods, along with their antioxidant levels, included: drinks, supplements, herbs, and spices, as well. Here are some foods that have high levels of antioxidants according to USDA research:

FRUIT: Including plums, sweet cherries, prunes, and apple types (like red delicious, granny smith, and gala apples).

BERRIES: Blueberries, raspberries, cranberries, strawberries, and blackberries all have high levels of antioxidants and can help you manage symptoms of your disorder.

BEANS: Dried beans like kidney, black, pinto, and red beans, are high in antioxidants levels, helping you fight off anxiety symptoms.

NUTS: Not only are nuts healthy for you in many ways, but they are also high in antioxidants. This is especially true of pecans and walnuts.

SPICES: Ginger and turmeric have both anti-anxiety and antioxidant properties and should be included in your diet.

VEGETABLES: Vegetables are great sources of antioxidants, including broccoli, beets, spinach, kale, and artichokes.

## Food effective in Combating anxiety

Anxiety disorders are among the most prevalent disorders worldwide, affecting 18 percent of the US population and 12 to 15 percent of the total population. Although most people suffering from anxiety seek treatment by taking Anxiety medications despite being aware of their multiple side effects and long-term use. But they feel they must go through this suffering and spend thousand on pharmaceuticals because it is the only option for them. Well, fortunately, that is not the case. Medicines and therapy are not the only way to treat anxiety. People suffering from anxiety can benefit a great deal if they include the following foods in their diet.

## Chamomile Tea

Chamomile tea is a natural medicine that works against anxiety and produces a calming effect on nerves. The soothing effect caused by this chamomile tea has been seen to effectively reduce anxiety and treat its symptoms to a great deal within a few days.

## Rooibos Tea

Rooibos is a tea that comes from the African Redbush. This delicious tea has shown remarkable results in calming nerves and treating anxiety. Studies conducted on its use in anxiety treatment have shown it to work on cortisol levels and reduce them. This tea's working mechanism balances stress and anxiety by bringing down the stress hormones in the body.

## Full-Fat Kefir

The gut is taken as a second brain the functional medicine because it contains almost 95 percent of the serotonin hormone that soothes the body and makes us feel good. Since the gut contains more than one hundred million neurons, the gut must be kept healthy to keep anxiety at bay.

Attacks by bacteria and viruses on your gut can seriously damage the serotonin neurons and cause anxiety. To prevent this from happening, Kefir, a unique fermented drink of dairy, can be used to provide a powerful defense against bacterial attack. It also contains some vitamins which keep the brain healthy such as A, D, K2 etc.

## Turmeric

Turmeric contains antioxidants in it called Curcuminoids that possess a protective quality for our nervous system and is good for elevating our mood. A study that used a random controlled method proved that turmeric effectively treats Depressive disorder and anxiety disorders.

## Avocados

Avocado is called a super fruit, which works wonders for our brain and helps reduce our anxiety levels. Avocadoes contain a great amount of Potassium, which automatically lower down our blood pressure. They also contain Vitamin B and saturated fats, which are very important for our brains' neurotransmitters.

## Dark Chocolate

Science has made it possible for cocoa lovers to indulge in their passion for chocolate without feeling guilty by proving its countless benefits. A study conducted on the link between chocolate and mood showed that people who drink more dark chocolate or eat dark chocolate are much more in control of their mood levels than other people. These people feel calmer and happier too.

## Asparagus

This vegetable contains many sulfur and vitamin B, folic acid, and many other beneficial ingredients. A low amount of folic acid has been linked with impairments of neurotransmitters, which cause anxiety. A serving of this food in 5.3 ounces increases the intake of folic acid by 60 percent. It also has potassium in it, which lowers the blood pressure naturally

## Apoptogenic Herbs

A very common Dysfunction in patients suffering from anxiety is in their Adrenal axis of Braun. The HPA axis is part of the fight or flight mechanism and manages the fatigue due to adrenal glands.

## Leafy Greens

People suffering from anxiety and stress should increase the intake of green veg in their diet. Foods like spinach and broccoli contain high magnesium, a chill pill that controls the brain's adrenal axis.

# ESSENTIAL OILS FOR ANXIETY RELIEF

Essential oils are the pure derivative of the plants they are extracted from. The result is a highly concentrated oil. Essential oils are a healthy and natural way to calm your body, mentally and physically. The molecules in the aroma of the oils can affect your brain and control stress and anxiety feelings. They also can change heart rate, blood pressure, and the function of your immune system.

How do essential oils help with anxiety?

When essential oils enter your body, they have incredible healing effects. The fragrance molecules from the oils travel through your olfactory system (one of the sensory systems responsible for your sense of smell) and make it to your brain to combat those feelings of anxiety and stress. Your limbic system is connected to certain parts of your brain that also affect blood pressure, hormone balance, and stress levels. Essential oils can be used topically or inhaled using aromatherapy to soothe anxiety. As outstanding healers, your body can absorb and spread its healing powers through your body within five minutes of exposure.

## Essential Oils for Anxiety and How to Use Them

### LAVENDER ESSENTIAL OIL

It is one of the most effective in treating anxiety. This oil can improve concentration, calm anger and irritability, and promote relaxation, which combats insomnia.

In my experience, there are a couple of ways to use lavender oil:

Topically: Place two to three drops on your wrists and rub them together, as if you were putting on perfume.

Use a diffuser: You can do this using an oil diffuser, which you can find at many stores and online.

In your bath: Run a hot bath and add a couple of drops of lavender to the water. While the steam from the warm bath will diffuse the oil and allow the soothing aroma to fill the room, your body will also absorb some of it while you are relaxing in the bath.

On your pillowcase: Put a couple of drops on your pillowcase so that you can let the aroma help you fall asleep and stay asleep.

### CEDARWOOD ESSENTIAL OIL

An essential oil that promotes serotonin release, which is a neurotransmitter in your body that regulates mood. Also, this oil helps regulate appetite. That is beneficial because, in some cases, feelings of anxiety can cause loss of appetite. Cedarwood oil also helps if you have trouble falling or staying asleep. In my experience, this oil also brings me feelings of confidence. This oil gives me a sense of power to overcome my stress and anxiety.

A couple of ways to use cedarwood oil:

As a massage lotion: Mix ¼ cup of coconut oil with twelve drops of cedarwood oil and add six orange essential oil drops. Massage into your feet, arms, and neck before bed and drift effortlessly to sleep.

As a moisturizer: Add a few drops of cedarwood oil to your favorite unscented body lotion or mix some drops with almond oil. Use these to moisturize your body as well as take advantage of its healing properties.

### EUCALYPTUS ESSENTIAL OIL

The strong aroma of this oil eliminates stress and gives you an energy boost. It is my favorite oil to use when I feel sluggish or mentally exhausted from stress and anxiety. It is the perfect pick-me-up to get rid of those feelings of sadness.

A couple of ways to use eucalyptus oil:

In your shower: Run a warm shower and plug the drain. Add three to five drops of eucalyptus oil to the water and let the warm water run over it. This will diffuse the oil and fill your shower with its refreshing aroma. You'll be ready to tackle anything that comes your way!

As an air freshener: Free your space from negative energy and use this oil as an air freshener. Simply mix twenty drops of eucalyptus oil with eight tablespoons of water in a spray bottle. Use this to bring positivity to any space, whether it be your bedroom, car, or office.

ROSE ESSENTIAL OIL

This oil is one of my favorites when I need an extra positivity boost. Also, this oil amps up my confidence because the aroma, to me, is very feminine. Rose oil also boosts feelings of peace and well-being.

A couple of ways to use rose oil:

After shower body spray: As a cherry on top after a refreshing shower, mix a few drops of rose oil with water in a spray bottle. Then, spray it in your hair, on your body, and even on your clothes to leave yourself feeling cleansed of all of those negative energies and stresses.

As a perfume: Rub two to three drops of rose oil on your wrists and neck for a confidence-boosting aroma to follow you throughout the day.

Essential oils are a powerful and versatile way to free your body from anxiety. The aromas and the properties of these oils are essential in your self-care recipe. In the next chapter, you will learn how meditation can rid your body and mind of anxiety. You will also learn how you can incorporate essential oils in your meditation practice for an extra soothing experience!

# DR. SEBI'S 3-STEP SOLUTION

Dr. Sebi's Official method for treating anxiety, such as any other disease, is composed of 3 main steps. Please note that any of these parts can't be passed over to succeed in your healing journey.

The three steps I'm talking about are:

1. Cleansing - The body must be cleaned on an intra-cellular level through detoxification to purify each cell and remove mucus excess.
2. Revitalizing - After cleansing, you need to nourish your body to regenerate your cells and strengthen the immune system.
3. Maintaining a Healthy Lifestyle- Follow Dr. Sebi's nutrition guide and adopt healthy lifestyle habits every day to keep your mind and body in good shape.

*Cleansing*

How to Prepare Cleansing Herbs?

Preparing your cleansing herbs would depend a lot on the form you purchased them. It's easier to prepare cleansing herbs in powder forms, as you can easily make herbal teas with them in the specified or recommended dosage. However, for other forms form herbs, especially roots or leaves, it is better to use a ratio of 1 teaspoon to 1 cup (8 oz) of spring water for each herb.

However, for easier batch preparation and storage, I recommend preparing herbs in batches of mixtures. That would mean mixing them up according to function and benefit. Again, this will depend on the state of your health and what minerals are most important for you. You can combine similar herbs with similar functions into a batch. Like our healer, Dr. Sebi would say: "If you want calcium, you know where to go to (sea moss), if you want Iron, you go to Burdock, and if you want a mix of both Iron and Fluorine, you go to Lily of the Valley".

In all, try not to mix more than 2 or 3 herbs. Remember, these herbs are electric, and it's best to preserve their organic carbon, hydrogen, and oxygen nature as much as we can. Again, if you mix more than that, you may not get their accurate concentrations per ml of water, so try to limit it to 3, possibly 2.

For a clearer understanding, you can use the following mix:

- Mix Colon and gallbladder cleansing herbs together
- Mix liver and kidney cleansing herbs
- Mix respiratory and mucus cleansing herbs
- Mix lymphatic and heavy-metal cleansing herbs.

Since these herbs perform a whole-body cleanse (not just colon), including the skin, eyes, colon, liver, lymphatic system, and gallbladder, you can decide to choose how to combine them. Also, note that when you make larger batches of these herbs for storage, try not to make batches that last more than 7 to 14 days.

For pre-purchase cleansing packages

Please follow the recommended dosage or instructions that are provided for that cleansing package

For fresh Green leafy herbs

- Place in spring water and boil on low heat for 5 to 7 min
- For dried leafy herbs, boil longer – 10 to 15 min

For Dried ground (or powder) herbs

For dried ground or powder leaves or roots, mix in recommended ratios for the herb. Powder herbs are the easiest to mix in dosage proportions, so you can simply follow the package instructions

For Chunks of Dried Root herbs

If you've purchased chunks of roots or stems, you can prepare them in the following way:

- Cut or break up chunks
- Place in spring water and boil for 15 minutes
- Let cool and serve
- Alternatively, prepare in larger batches and place in jars to store in the refrigerator.

For bulk purchase herbs

If you have purchased herbs in bulk and you're making your teas, find out what the recommended dosage is for each herb. As a general rule, you should prepare each herbal tea ratio of 1 teaspoon to 8 ounces of spring water.

For capsules

I recommend that you do research and find out what the recommended dosage is for each herbal capsule

How To Take The Prepared Cleansing Herbs

If you are on medication, I recommend taking the herbs one hour before taking your meds; Dr. Sebi recommended this. Your colon cleansing herbs should not be consumed for longer than 30 days because your body may become dependent on them, and you want to start to reduce the dose during your last 3 to 5 days, depending on how long you've been taking them.

Routine:

- Twice a day - morning and night
- Daily Consistency - Try to stay consistent both in terms of timing and duration. That is, try not to skew the duration. Make it consistent, and take the cleansing herb throughout the cleanse. For example, for a 14-day cleanse, the cleansing herbs can be taken twice daily, and you should take them around the same time you do take them on both mornings and evenings.
- Gradual Wean Off – Just like medications, it is not the best to go cold-turkey when it comes to herbal detox. Towards the end of the cleanse duration, wean off your herbs by gradually reducing the dosage and duration. The duration of the wean will depend on the length of the fast you choose. For example, for a one month fast, I usually start weaning a week towards closure. For a 14 day fast, I begin weaning on day 11 or 12. You can begin the wean by reducing it from twice a day to once a day. Or simply take half the dosages each for mornings and night.

You must do this because you need to signal your body to begin to prepare to start functioning independently without dependence on herbs' cleansing. And no other way to do this than to take it slow and gradual, without bringing too much "shock" to your body.

How to break a detox fast?

- Slowly reintroduce solids

If you are doing water or a liquid fast, you will need to reintroduce solid foods slowly. You can begin by introducing solids like high water-content fruits. These include watermelon, apples, and berries. After that, you can proceed to introduce softer fruit solids like bananas and avocados. Later, you can incorporate more harder solids like veggies. All foods must be listed on the nutrition guide. However, if doing a fruit or raw veggie fast, you can break the fast right away on solid foods.

- Drink 1-gallon spring water daily

Drink spring water daily together with the revitalizing herbs and sea moss.

How long should you detox/cleanse?

How long you should detox depends on your state of health, that is, your body's toxification level (the less healthy you are, the more toxic your body is) and tolerance level. Typically, it is recommended to fast for 7-14 days, but Dr. Sebi recommends a minimum of at least a 12 day fast. Dr. Sebi himself fasted for 90 days to cure himself of diabetes, asthma, and impotence. It is great to cleanse at least once a year for seven days if you consume an alkaline diet. If you are not consuming an alkaline diet, then you should cleanse/detox every three months

I fasted for 14 days, and I would recommend fasting for between 14 days and one month if you have high blood pressure. Again, your body's tolerance level will ultimately determine the length so, watch your body and study its reaction as you begin the fast. We are all different, and you may find that you cannot handle a basic liquid fast (water or juice). In that case, you can get started with fruit or raw vegetables fast. But make sure all foods and fruits are listed in the Dr. Sebi Nutrition Guide. Whether liquid, juice, or raw food fast, the results are virtually all the same – the only major difference is when it takes to begin to see results. While raw food fasts take longer, liquid fasts are much faster. So do not worry; the most important thing is to stay committed and focused on whatever fasting method you choose.

Common Symptoms Expected During Detox Cleanse

- Cold and Flu symptoms
- Changes in Bowel movements
- Fatigue and Low Energy
- Difficulty sleeping
- Itching
- Headaches
- Muscle aches and pains
- Acne. Rashes and breakouts
- Mucus expel (catarrh, etc.)
- Lower blood pressure

If you relate to any of these symptoms during the cleansing stage, be happy. That's because your body is pushing out all the toxins and mucus you have been keeping inside for so long. These symptoms are only temporary and usually resolve after the first one to two weeks.

## HERBS TO TAKE DURING DETOX

Below are listed the herbs Dr. Sebi recommended to use to cleanse your body and relieve anxiety symptoms:

### Cascara Sagrada

It is a natural laxative, purgative shrub plant from Rhamnaceae's family that Dr. Sebi recommended because of its potency to causes muscle contractions in the intestine, detox/cleanse the colon, stimulate liver and pancreas secretion, and moves stool through the bowel. This herb is rich in glycosides, Vitamin-A, B, C, and D, emodin, and anthracoid, making it very effective in cleansing and revitalizing herbs.

The benefits of Consuming Cascara Sagrada include:

- It helps to get rid of toxins from the colon.
- It serves as a laxative for constipation.
- It helps to soothe and dissolve gallstones.
- It helps to treat and prevent liver problems.
- It helps to destroy and inhibit cancerous cells from mutation.
- It helps to soothe and treats digestive problems.
- It relieves joint and muscle pain and other pains that are caused by inflammation.
- It treats transmitted diseases caused by viruses and bacterial

When writing this book, there are no side effects attributed to healthy adults who have to consume Cascara sagrada for a short period.

The note-full precautions before Consuming Cascara Sagrada are:

- Nursing mothers should avoid these herbs because they can inflict their baby with diarrhea.
- If you suffer from disease or health disorders like; stomach irritation or upset without knowing the cause, any colitis, kidney disorders, intestinal blockage, or Crohn's disease, please do not use this herb without medical supervision.

For the dosage and how to prepare cascara sagrada tea, kindly take the steps below:

1. Get Cascara Sagrada plants and remove some of the bark, and chopped it.
2. Once you have chopped it, dry it until it is dried, or you can order it online, and it will come chopped and dried.
3. Pour 8-10 ounces of water into your saucepan and add 1-1½ teaspoon of cascara sagrada bark in the saucepan.
4. Steams the mixture for 15-20 minutes on your cooker.
5. After the 15-20 minutes, steam, allow it to reduce its hotness, and strain it to remove the chopped bark of cascara sagrada.
6. You are done. For the dosage, consume 1 cup (8-10 ounce) of Cascara Sagrada tea 2-3 times daily.

## Rhubarb Root

Rhubarb Root is a very effective laxative that Dr. Sebi recommended because of its effectiveness in boosting the digestive tract's health. However, Rhubarb roots are very rich with various nutrients, making it a perfect herb for cleansing the body.

The benefits of Consuming Rhubarb Root are:

- It helps to treat various types of sores like; canker sores, cold sores, etc.
- It helps to destroy various types of viruses like; herpes simplex virus, HIV, etc.
- It helps to enhance and relieve the symptoms of menopause.
- It helps to serve as a remedy for the treatment of pancreatitis (swelling of the pancreas).
- It helps boost and enhance people's respiratory system suffering from ARDS to enable them to breathe healthier.
- It helps to soothe and cure menstrual pain (dysmenorrhea).
- It helps to treat and stop blood bleeding in the stomach.
- It helps to treat and prevent gastrointestinal (GI) bleeding.
- It helps to shed excess body weight (cholesterol) naturally.

When writing this book, there are no side effects attributed to consuming Rhubarb root and its rhizome for over two years, except it leaves that contain oxalic acid, which is unsafe.

For the dosage and how to prepare Rhubarb root tea, kindly take the steps below:

1. Uproot some root of Rhubarb plant (make sure that the plants uprooted are above four years, and it is in autumn).

2. Wash the uprooted roots under running water to remove all dirt that accompanied it from the soil and remove the external fibers, and dried it on a plane surface.

3. Once it is dried, chopped it into smaller pieces. (Not more than 0.5 inch) or pound it and stored it in a tightly closed container. Alternatively, you can order it online, and it will come dried and chopped.

4. Pour 8 ounces of water in a saucepan and add 1tablespoon of the pounded or chopped rhubarb root, and boil the mixture for 15-20minutes v. After the timing, reduced the heat of the gas for about 10 minutes and put off the fire.

5. Allow it to get cold for at least 10-15minute and strain out the root.

6. You are done. For the dosage, take 1 cup (8ounce) of the infusion three times per day.

## *Ashwagandha*

The benefits of using or consuming Ashwagandha also include:

- It helps to reduce stress fast by regulating chemicals in your brain
- It is widely used to fight anxiety in herbal medicine
- Being an energy booster, it helps not to feel fatigued
- It may help improve heart health by reducing cholesterol and triglyceride levels
- It may help to reduce sugar levels in people suffering from diabetes
- It acts as a pain reliever, preventing pain signals from traveling along the central nervous system.
- May increase muscle mass and muscle strength

Dosage and administration:

Take 250mg to 3000mg daily with abundant water at the morning.

## Mullein

Mullein is a flavorful beverage flowering plant that has been used for centuries to treat various ailments. Research shows that this herb is an effective anti-microbial, anti-inflammatory, anti-cancer, anti-hepatotoxic, antioxidant, and anti-viral herb with potency to prevent a lot of health disorders. It helps to cleanse and detoxify the lungs and lymph system and destroy cancer.

The benefits of consuming Mullein include:

- It helps treat and prevent various types of cancer by destroying cancerous cells and preventing them from mutating.
- It helps to eliminate mucus from the small intestine
- It helps to activate healthy lymph circulation in the chest and neck
- It helps neutralize the negatives effects of free radicals by protecting the cells from damages caused by free radicals.
- It helps treat and prevent various bacterial and virus infections like herpes viruses, HIV etc.
- It helps to treat and prevent respiratory tract infections.
- It helps to treat and prevent tuberculosis.
- It helps to treat earache.
- It helps to treat various health disorders like bronchitis, stroke, heart diseases etc.
- It helps to prevent some chronic brain diseases like Alzheimer's, Parkinson's etc.

- It helps to treat atherosclerosis and others in the biological systems.
- It helps to treat and relieve pain that is caused by inflammation and tumor.
- It also helps treat various ailments like asthma, bronchitis, migraine, congestion etc.

When writing this book, there are no negative side effects attributed to mullein consumption by mouth; But, since there is no information to show that this herb is harmful or not to pregnant and breastfeeding mothers, I advise them to avoid its consumption.

When writing this book, there are no medications that interact with mullein as it can be combined with other herbs and drugs without any issues.

For the dosage and how to prepare Mullein tea, kindly take the steps below:

1. Harvest some fresh mullein leaves, dry it until it is dried and chopped it into smaller pieces. Alternatively, you can place an order online, and it will come dried and chopped.
2. Once the fresh leaves are dried, measure 1-2 teaspoon and pour it into your teacup or mug.
3. Measure 8-10 ounces of water and boil it.
4. Once the water is boiling, pour it inside your teacup or mug where the mullein leaves are and allow it to steep for 15-20 minutes.
5. Strain it, and you are done!
6. For the dosage, take 1 cup (8-10ounce) 2-3 times daily.

## German Chamomile

The benefits of consuming German Chamomile include:

- It helps to treat and calm the central nervous system.
- It helps to treat and prevent swelling (inflammation)
- It helps to boost the functionalities of the brain and heal the brain.
- It helps serves as a laxative that helps to enhance healthy sleep and relieve depression.
- It helps to relieve and soothe stomach and intestine cramps and soothe indigestion (dyspepsia).
- It helps to shed excess body fat by reducing cholesterol in the body.
- It helps treat and prevent skin disorders like eczema, etc., and cold and flu.

The note-full precautions before consuming German Chamomile are:

- Because there is no much information regarding whether German Chamomile is harmful to pregnant and breast-feeding mothers or not, I advise that they stay off this herb completely.
- People that are allergic to plant from Asteraceae/Compositae family should stay off German Chamomile.
- Because German Chamomile increases estrogen, people suffering from; hormone-sensitive disorder like; breast, uterine and ovarian cancer, uterine fibroid, endometriosis, etc., should stay off this herb.

For the dosage and how to prepare German Chamomile, kindly take the steps below:

1. Get some fresh flowers of German chamomile and dry it in a plane surface
2. Once it is dried, pound it into smaller pieces, or you can order it online, and it will come dried and chopped.

3. Boil 10 ounces of water.
4. Measure 1-2 teaspoons of the dried flower of German chamomile and pour it into your teacup/ mug.
5. Pour the boiled water into the teacup/mug, cover it and allow it to steep for 10-15 minutes.
6. Filter it using a filter and pressed the marc to get the new active principle inside the cell.
7. You are done. Take 1 cup (100ounce) of the tea/infusion 1 time per day before eating anything for the dosage.

## Valerian Root

The benefits of consuming valerian roots include:

- It helps treat and calm the central nervous system, relieve anxiety, stress, depression, and chronic fatigue syndrome (CFS).
- It helps to treat and prevent sleeplessness (Insomnia).
- It helps relieve and reduces the severity and frequency of hot flashes in postmenopausal women and relief premenstrual disorders (PMS).
- It helps to soothe dysmenorrhea (menstrual cramps) and relieve pains during menstruation.
- It may help to lower blood pressure and the rate of heartbeat.
- It is used to remedy Attention-deficit hyperactivity disorder (ADHD).
- It is used to treat and relieve some health issues like: headache, convulsions, epilepsy, mild tremor, joint pains, stomach irritation, etc.

Valerian root has no side effects if used for less than 28 days, but if you consume too much of it, you might suffer some side effects like:

- Stomach irritation.
- Headache
- Swing mood
- Sleeplessness
- Sluggishness

The note-full precautions before consuming valerian root include:

- Since much is unknown about this herb's safety for pregnant and breastfeeding mothers, I advise them to stay off this herb.
- Because of this herb's drowsiness effect, I strongly advise you not to drive or operate any machinery after consuming valerian root.

For the dosage and how to prepare Valerian root tea, kindly take the following steps:

1. Harvest some valerian plants' roots, wash them, chop them into smaller pieces, and dried them.
2. Alternatively, you can order it online, and it will come dried and chopped.
3. Boil 8-10 ounces of water and add 1teaspoon of the valerian root and allow it to boil for 15-20 minutes.
4. Allow it to get cool and strain.
5. You are done! For the dosage, take 1 cup (8-100ounce) of valerian tea 30-60minutes before going to bed daily.

## Dandelion

Dandelion is a flowering plant known as 'yellow gowan' or 'lion's tooth'. This plant is native to Eurasia and today. It is common in over 60 countries worldwide in the mild climates of the northern hemisphere. For centuries, these flowering plants have been used for the treatment of swelling (inflammation) of the pancreas, relieve pains that are caused by inflammation, treat and prevent cancer, tonsils (tonsillitis), skin disorder, bladder or urethra disorder, digestive and liver problems and enhance the general health of the liver and digestive system.

Researchers proved that it is a very effective cleansing/detoxification herbs because of the chemical compositions and nutrients.

The benefits of using or consuming Dandelion include:

- It helps to detoxify or cleanse the liver and the kidney.
- It helps to treat and prevent diabetes by regulating blood sugar levels.
- It helps to fight against and relieve pains that are caused by inflammation.
- It helps to deactivate and inhibit the negative effects of free radicals in the body, which is because of its antioxidant properties.
- It reduces the level of cholesterol.
- It lowers blood pressure by getting rid of excess fluid in the body.
- It helps to naturally shed excess weight gain by improving the metabolism of carbohydrates.
- It helps in boosting the digestive system.
- It helps to boost the immune system.
- It helps to keep the skin healthy and treat and prevent skin diseases.

Till at the time of writing this book, Dandelion is 100% safe, but consuming an overdose of it can result in some side effects like:

- Experiencing stomach upset or irritation
- Allergic reactions

The special precautions before using/consuming dandelions are:

- Pregnant and breastfeeding mothers should stay off dandelion as there is no research to know if it is harmful to them or not.
- If you are suffering from Eczema, stays off dandelion as more than 85% of people with eczema suffer an allergic reaction to dandelion.

For the dosage and how to prepare Dandelion tea/infusion, kindly take the following steps:

1. Get some fresh leaves of dandelion and washed it under running water to remove all the dirt.
2. After washing it, pour ½ - 1 cup of the washed dandelion into your saucepan.
3. You should boil 4-5 cups of water and pour the boiled water inside the saucepan where you pour the dandelion and cover it for 12-15 hours or throughout the night (overnight).
4. The next day, strain out the dandelion leaves, and you will be left with the dandelion tea/infusion.
5. For the dosage, take ½ tablespoon of Dandelion per ¾ cup of water three times daily. And if

you ordered your dandelion online, you can take 4-10 grams of dry leaf of dandelion three times daily.

## Prodigiosa

Prodigiosa, also known as 'Prodijiosa or Hamula, is a perennial plant with large bushy leaves and flowers, and it's from the daisy family and native to Mexico and California. These plants have a grey-purple hue on the underside and dark green leaves on the upper side and grow up to 5 feet in height with its flowers growing in clusters. This plant has a long history with the Mexicans as it has been used for centuries to treat diabetes, arthritis, diarrhea, and stomach disorder and relieve aching joints.

Because of the chemical and compound composition of Prodigiosa, research has it that it is very effective for the treatment of diabetes II because of how it aids in stimulating the pancreatic gland to secret and reduces or lowers blood sugar level and burn down fat in the gallbladder. The irony is that Prodigiosa can cause more damage to people that are suffering from Type I diabetes. Furthermore, consuming Prodigiosa's tea/infusion helps boost the digestion of fat and improve the synthesis of bile in the liver, dissolve tiny gallstones, and treat chronic gastritis and other digestive systems disorders. Although there is no research to prove its effectiveness in treating cataracts, it is believed that it can cure cataracts.

Prodigiosa is used for several reasons, included:

- Treatment of diabetes (type II).
- Treatment of diarrhea.
- Treatment of stomach pain.
- Treatment of gallbladder disease.
- Enhancing the digestion of fat and boosting the digestive system's healthiness.

The note-full precautions to beware of before using or consuming Prodigiosa includes:

- Pregnant and breastfeeding mothers should not use or consume Prodigiosa as there is no research to back it if it is safe or not.
- It is a no-go area for people suffering from diabetes I., and people with diabetes II should control their sugar level while consuming this herb.

How to prepare Prodigiosa tea/infusion:

1. Dry the fresh leaves until it is dried.
2. Once the fresh leaves are dried, or the one you ordered for is available, boil eight or 16ounce of water and brew 1 or 2 tablespoons of Prodigiosa leaves in the warm water for 15minutes.
3. After brewing it, strain the Prodigiosa leaves.
4. Take a cup (8ounce) of Prodigiosa tea/infusion two times per day for the dosage.

## Burdock Root

Burdock root is the root of a delicious plant called Burdock, which all its body or parts are useful as either food or medicine. This plant can be found all over the world. I called this plant the wonder plant because everything about it is important as we consume its root as food, and we also use it for medicinal purposes, and both its leaf and seed are used for medicinal purposes.

For over five centuries, people worldwide have been using burdock root orally to treat and prevent various health disorders.

Because of Burdock root's chemical composition, such as; quercetin and luteolin, research has it that it can serve as a great effective antioxidants that can treat and prevent cancer by preventing cancerous cells from growing and mutating and also combat aging. Compound like 'Phytosterols' helps boost scalp and hair follicles to grow healthy hair even from baldhead. The vitamins-C helps in boosting the immune system and combat bacterial. It also helps to cleanse or detoxify the liver and lymphatic system, etc.

The potassium helps reduce blood sugar levels and filter the blood by removing impurities through the bloodstream and eradicating toxins through the skin and urine.

The benefits of using or consuming burdock root tea/infusion include:

- cleanse/detox the liver and lymphatic system.
- Treat and prevent diabetes by reducing blood sugar levels in the body.
- Eliminate toxins from the body by inducing sweetness and urine.
- Purify the blood by removing heavy metals from the bloodstream.
- Treat various skin disorders and combat aging.
- Treat and prevent cancer by inhibiting the growth and mutation of cancerous cells.
- Boost the immune system and enhance circulation.

Till at the time of writing this book, there are no side effects that have been recorded by researchers or people that have used these herbs.

However, research has it that applying this root to your skin might cause rashes.

For the dosage and how to prepare Burdock root tea/infusion, kindly take the following steps:

1. Scrub the uprooted root of burdock heartily under running water to remove all the dirt that accompanied it from the soil.
2. You should chop the Burdock root into smaller pieces (less than 1 inch). Please note that if you order it online, it will come dried and already chopped.
3. Pour 2-3 cup of water into your saucepan and add ¼ cup of the chopped burdock root and boil it.
4. Once the water is boiling, lower your gas, re-boil it for 30-40 minutes, and put off your gas.
5. Once it is cold, strain it and consume it.
6. For the dosage, drink one glass cup daily

## Revitalizing

Below are listed the herbs Dr. Sebi recommended to use for revitalizing your body's cells and fight anxiety:

## Irish Sea Moss

Irish Sea Moss is red algae that belong to the family of Florideophytes that grows on the rocky parts of the Atlantic coast of various countries, including the British Isles, Jamaica, Scotland, etc. Dr. Sebi recommends this herb for revitalizing the body after cleansing because it has over 92 out of 102 minerals that the body needs to be healthy. Some minerals are, for example:

- Phosphorus
- Iodine
- Selenium
- Calcium
- Bromine
- Iron
- Potassium

Some of the benefits of consuming Irish Sea Moss are:

- It heal and boost the immune defense system.
- It treats and prevents hyperthyroidism and boosts the functionalities and health of the thyroid.
- It helps to soothe joint pain and swelling of the joint and treat arthritis.
- It helps to enrich the overall mood and reduce fussiness.
- It helps to combat infections caused by viruses and bacterial.
- It helps treat and prevent various skin disorders like acne, skin wrinkling, and alleviating inflammation.
- It helps to treat and prevent digestive and respiratory tract disorders.

The note-full precautions to beware of before consuming Irish Sea moss include:

- Because of how rich Irish Sea moss is with iron, it can trigger hypothyroidism for people suffering from Hashimoto's disease.
- Stop using the herb if you notice any allergies or reactions.

For the dosage and how to prepare Irish Sea Moss tea, kindly take the steps below:

- Measure and boil 1cups (8ounce) of water in a ceramic pot.
- Once the water is boiled, measure 2-3 tablespoon of Irish Sea moss gel (or 1teaspoon for the fine form) and add it to the boiling water.
- Allow the Irish Sea moss for 10-15 minutes to dissolve completely.

You are done!

For the dosage, take 1cup of Irish Sea moss tea daily in the morning.

## Sensitiva

Also known as 'Mimosa pudica', which is of the Fabaceae family, is a species that is native to Central and South America. However, it is currently spread in other tropical regions and is gaining popularity among many people worldwide as a medicinal herb.

Besides being a fun, intriguing element of nature, Sensitive plant is also filled with many health benefits.

The health benefits of consuming Sensitiva herb are:

- It helps cure joint pain and arthritis

- It treats insomnia and sleeplessness
- It treats Asthma
- It helps to cure gum problems and toothaches
- It fights hair loss
- It lowers blood sugar level and help who suffers from diabetes
- It lowers high blood pressure
- It helps to treat stomachaches

Dosage and administration:

Liquid: Dose about 3 to 6 ml of 1:2 mimosa liquid extract daily

Capsule: 1 tablet, three times daily with meals

However, capsule and liquid extract formulations are proprietary herbal blends and are available in several strength.

## Soursop

Soursop is the fruit of the "Annona Muricata" tree that is a native of tropical regions in the Americas that belongs to the Annonaceae family. Its leaves are widely used because they are rich with various nutrients like iron, calcium, phosphorus, magnesium, sodium, potassium, zinc, etc. That makes the tea very effective in fighting against the mutation of cancerous cells.

Other benefits of consuming soursops tea are:

- It helps to destroy and eliminate cancerous cells and inhibit the growth of cancer cells.
- It is a very strong and effective antioxidant that helps neutralize free radicals that can damage the cells.
- It helps to soothe heart disorders.
- It helps to lower blood sugar levels for people who have type 2 diabetes.
- It helps to fight against infectious diseases caused by bacterial. Such diseases like: yeast infections, cholera, gingivitis, Staphylococcus, tooth decay etc.
- It helps to soothe and alleviates swelling (inflammation) etc.

The note-full precautions before consuming of soursops tea include:

- Since there is no information about this herb's harmful effects on pregnant and breastfeeding mothers, I advise that they stay off this herb.
- Although this herb is tempting, please make sure you consume this herb under a medical practitioner's supervision.

For the dosage and how to prepare soursops tea, kindly take the following steps:

- Harvest some fresh Soursops leaves, dry it until it is dried, chop it, or pound it into smaller pieces. On the other hand, you can place an order online, and it will come dried and chopped.
- Measure one teaspoon of the chopped leaves of the Soursops and pour it into your teacup or mug.
- Boil 8 ounces of water and add it to the Soursop leaves in the teacup or mug and cover it.
- Allow the leaves to steep for 10-15 minutes and strain it.

You are done!

For the dosage, consume 2-3 cups of Soursops tea daily.

## Cordoncillo Negro

The cordincillo negro is a shrub whose leaves give off a spicy smell when squeezed and a bitter taste when chewed.

Cordoncillo negro has many important uses.

For example:

- It can be used as a painkiller. Chewing on the leaves of cordoncillo anesthetizes the mouth. If you squeeze and rub these leaves over a cut or wound it can serve as an anesthetic.
- It can treat digestion problems like vomiting, nausea, stomach ache, dyspepsia, dysentery, etc.
- It can also prevent blood loss from internal bleeding
- It can treat respiratory problems like colds, flu, coughs, bronchitis, and pneumonia.
- Helps to keep the kidney healthy and prevent kidney stones

Dosage and administration:

Infusion: 1 cup 2-3 times daily

## Blue Vervain

Blue Vervain is a perennial flowering plant that belongs to the family of Verbenaceae. It is rich with various nutrients like iron fluorine, which purifies the blood, phosphorus, phosphate, zinc, potassium, magnesium, etc. Because of this potency, Dr. Sebi recommends this herb for revitalizing your body after cleansing.

The benefits of using or consuming Blue Vervain include:

- It helps to treat and prevent anxiety and sleeplessness and enhance mood.
- It helps to treat and calm the central nervous system.
- It helps to soothe the nerves and relaxes the mind, thereby treating migraine headaches.
- It helps boost and protect the heart's health, treat and prevent myocardial ischemia, chest pain, and heart failure.
- It helps to fight against both internal and external inflammation.
- It helps to treat menstrual cramps or pain and stomach pain.
- It improves digestive health and protects the livers and kidneys by cleansing/detoxifying both the kidney and liver.

The note-full precautions before consuming of soursops tea include:

- Because there is no information to show if these herbs are good for breastfeeding mothers or pregnant women, I advise that they avoid these herbs' consumption.
- Till at the time of writing this book, there are no medications that interact with blue Vervain.

For the dosage and how to prepare Blue Vervain tea, kindly take the following steps:

1. Get some fresh leaves and flowers of blue Vervain and dry them.

2. Once it is dried, pound or chopped it, or you can order it online, and it will come dried and chopped.
3. Boil a cup of water (8ounce) in a saucepan.
4. Once the water is boiled, pour it into a cup, measure 1 teaspoon of the Blue Vervain, and add it to the water.
5. Allow it to steep for 10-15 minutes and strain it.
6. You are done! For the dosage, take 2-4 cups daily.

When Should I Consume the Revitalizing Herbs?

The best time to consume the revitalizing herbs is the next day after you finish your cleanse. For instance, if you fast for 14days, on the 15day, you should start consuming your revitalizing herbs.

What Are the Things That I Shouldn't Forget?

- Drink at least a gallon of spring water daily.
- Once you are done with your detox /cleanse, eat foods only on Dr. Sebi's nutritional guide.
- Never forget to use sea moss
- Ensure you do an intra-cellular cleanse once per year for at least seven days if you follow only the alkaline diet from Dr. Sebi's nutritional guide. Still, if you are not, you should always do an intra-cellular cleansing after every three months to cleanse your body from mucus and toxins.

Please note that consuming acidic food can only put your body at the risk of relapsing.

Maintaining a Healthy Lifestyle

## Dieting

Nope, this isn't the latest fad diet to help you lose weight! Dieting for anxiety is about eating healthily. As mentioned above, the food we eat has a direct (often fast-acting) impact on our mood and emotional state. A balanced, healthy diet is essential for good physical health, a stable, healthy weight, and mental health.

Healthy diets should include a balance of low-fat protein sources and lots of fruits and vegetables.

There are several food types that you may need to avoid if you suffer from anxiety:

- High sugar foods boost our energy levels quickly but may promote adrenaline production, which causes feelings of anxiety.
- Processed foods; often contain high levels of sugar and a range of other additives, which will potentially imbalance the chemicals in your brain, leading to more or more severe panic episodes.
- Caffeine; as mentioned above, caffeine gives a boost, and one cup is usually OK. However, in excess, it will promote imbalances in your brain chemistry, over-stimulating adrenaline production and leading to high levels of anxiety.
- Alcohol: long term misuse of alcohol can lead to developing anxiety disorders. It's also often a symptom of the conditions and those suffering from depression related illnesses. Cutting alcohol consumption is strongly recommended but seeking help to do so is also wise.

Some foods are better for us than others and, when it comes to brain food, certain types of food can have a profound effect on our mood. The following food types have been identified as having positive effects on our brain's functions and chemistry.

For those with anxiety-related disorders, incorporating them into your diet is a must:

- Vitamin B is essential for good physical health, and it also helps to regulate mood. Sources include vitamin supplements, citrus fruits and leafy green vegetables,
- Another essential is Omega-3; this, as with vitamin B, helps regulate mood and has several positive physical effects. It's found mostly in oily fish, but you can find them in dried fruits too. As part of a healthy balanced diet, you should aim to consume at least two to three portions per week.

## Exercise

Exercise has been clinically proven to reduce anxiety and improve mood and it can also treat many other health problems. Health issues can be a major anxiety trigger, but easing the symptoms of those ailments can further reduce anxiety.

When a person exercises, their body always releases hormones that produce a calming effect and increases body temperature, which can be very relaxing. Working up a sweat is tiring, but it's a great way to calm down.

When some people hear the word "exercise," they picture a gym full of lifting weights. However, many fitness activities can provide the exercise someone with anxiety needs. Even everyday activities like gardening or washing a car can elevate the mood.

Many people think they don't have time for exercise, but exercise doesn't have to take hours. Instead, people can find little ways to increase physical activity throughout the day. They might stretch at their desk at work or take a quick walk during their lunch break.

Studies suggest that 30 minutes of exercise a day, three days a week can dramatically reduce anxiety symptoms. However, those same studies show that even small amounts of activity can have a positive effect. If someone doesn't have time for lengthy workouts, they should still find ways to exercise their body needs.

While increase physical activity provides several health benefits, they aren't lasting. For exercise to improve anxiety, it must be done consistently. That makes it all the more important for people to find exercise routines they can stick with and physical activities that they enjoy.

For many people who suffer from anxiety, beginning an exercise routine is the hardest part. However, once they get started, they find these physical activity periods to be one of the most enjoyable parts of the day. Sticking with an exercise routine can be very easy if that routine is planned out well.

Anyone beginning an exercise routine should think about the physical activities they enjoy most. Do they enjoy playing with their children? Riding a bicycle? Gardening in their backyard? When it comes to reducing anxiety symptoms, any activity that gets the body moving counts as exercise.

No one should feel as though they have to decide on a workout plan and stick to it forever. Sampling a variety of different activities can help keep motivation levels high. Different kinds of exercises have different benefits, and switching between them gives people the chance to experience them all.

If the thought of joining a gym is enough to bring on a panic attack – you're probably not alone. You don't need to have a social phobia (or any other kind of anxiety disorder) to have an aversion to the gym! However, healthy exercise has some surprising implications for anxiety disorders and other psychological conditions, including depression. The mechanisms by which exercise and mental health are related are not fully understood. Many medical experts worldwide now acknowledge that exercise has a major impact on a wide range of psychological conditions. It is believed that exercise can be as effective at combating depression as many commonly prescribed drugs.

Moderate level intensity exercise is recommended as perfect for improving your physical health and also your mental health. That includes walking briskly, cycling, jogging, or swimming. Walking and jogging should not need any investment, and if you're uncomfortable alone, partner up with a friend or relative. Ideally, buddy up with someone who addresses the same issues or has a good understanding of them for extra support.

Psychologists recommend that the exercises you choose should be rhythmic and repetitive. That helps to clear the mind and focus it on the task at hand. Walking, again, is the simplest of these and should be easy to achieve for many people.

If you find that you begin to experience anxiety during a period of exercise, simply focus your mind on your breathing. Use a meditation technique like "mindfulness meditation" (described briefly in the next chapter) to become aware of your body, breathing simply, and limiting the impact of negative or nervous thoughts. Experience the moment that you are in, not the fears that are in your mind. Alternatively, simply count each step (out-loud if necessary) to distract your mind from the feelings of anxiety.

## Good Sleep Does the Trick

When you don't get good sleep, you drain your entire body and brain of vital functioning energy. In response, your body and brain are reduced to anxiety; it may be hard for you to focus and make logical thoughts. On the other hand, anyone experiencing an anxiety episode is advised to get a maximum of 8 hours of uninterrupted sleep. I know I say 8 hours, and it may be hard even to make them fall asleep. What you can do, try and prepare the environment in which they will sleep in, make it cozy, warm, and secure; you can even sleep by their side so that they know you are there. When you do all these, the person's brain starts adjusting from anxiety mode to relief mode, and thoughts like, 'I think I am safe in this room, I think she will make me safe' is what will be crossing their minds.

## Teas

Tea has the power to relieve anxiety on some levels. The very act of drinking tea is relaxing, particularly when that tea is hot. It also requires people to take a few minutes to sit and relax, which anxiety sufferers need badly.

It creates a positive routine, which is relaxing in and of itself. Studies have shown that following calming routines can play a role in reducing anxiety symptoms. Also, tea provides the body with the hydration it needs to fight back against anxiety symptoms.

However, the real benefit of teas comes from the herbs they contain. Many herbs found in tea can provide long-term anxiety relief. Drinking tea made from fresh herbs can have a particularly beneficial effect, but even packaged tea can be quite helpful.

One type of tea that is particularly good at easing tension is valerian root. This herb is a natural sedative and can help the body to process emotions more effectively. It works particularly well for people who are unable to get enough sleep because of their anxiety. However, it should be noted that this tea could cause some people to feel lethargic.

Research has shown that blue vervain can calm the nervous system and effectively treat many nervous conditions. It can also help people get a more restful night's sleep. However, even though this tea works very well, experts recommend against drinking it regularly. It's better for occasional relief.

You can also use Chamomile Tea. Chamomile tea is famous for its ability to aid in relaxation. It soothes many anxiety symptoms and can also calm a nervous stomach. People who have experienced a reduction in appetite because of their stress should give chamomile a try. It may provide them with anxiety relief while restoring their appetite.

One of the advantages of chamomile is that children can safely consume this tea. Many children suffer from anxiety, and this natural relief method can help them cope with their symptoms. However, when it comes to people under the age of twelve, it's recommended that chamomile not be taken for an extended period.

Another type of tea that you can also use is Lemon Balm Tea. Lemon balm tea works to soothe the nervous system, reducing feelings of anxiety and stress. It also has the power to relieve headaches, which are commonly experienced by people with anxiety disorders. Those who don't enjoy hot tea can experience lemon balm tea's soothing properties by drinking it iced.

Green tea is also another type of tea that you can use to help treat your anxiety as long as you drink decaffeinated tea. Most green tea contains caffeine, which means that many anxiety sufferers often avoid it. However, it also contains a substance called theanine, which promotes alpha waves in the brain. This can provide a significant amount of relaxation. Decaffeinated green tea allows people to reap theanine benefits while avoiding the negative side effects of caffeine.

Tea can ease the symptoms of anxiety on some levels. It's a good idea for anxiety sufferers to experiment with different teas, as this allows them to see which types provide them with the most relief. Some teas are more effective when taken daily, while others should only be taken on occasion.

Tea is healthy, calming, and can benefit the mind and body in several ways. It's more than a beverage; it's a potent way to treat health problems and reduce stress. Tea should be a part of any anxiety sufferer's life.

### Acupuncture

For years, Western people have approached acupuncture with skepticism. They didn't understand how sticking needles into the body could relieve anxiety symptoms. Many people thought that the practice of acupuncture should cause people to experience more anxiety.

It's easy to see why people have such a hard time wrapping their heads around the concept of acupuncture. Acupuncture is based on the ancient Chinese principle of qi. Proponents of acupuncture believe that correctly balancing qi in the body can cure several ailments. While qi's concept hasn't been sufficiently studied, recent research has helped prove that acupuncture can provide anxiety relief. More importantly, it has been discovered why it's so effective.

When the body is stressed, some hormones are secreted. These hormones affect the pituitary gland and the adrenal gland and cause many of the symptoms most commonly associated with anxiety. These hormones can also trigger the " fight or flight" response, leading to panic attacks.

However, acupuncture can block these stress-induced hormone elevations. It can change the way blood circulates in the body and can improve overall nerve function. Study after study has demonstrated that acupuncture works.

Although acupuncture was once considered alternative medicine, its increased legitimacy has led to acupuncture treatments being covered by several insurance companies. This allows many people to take advantage of one of the most effective anxiety treatments available.

It is important to note that acupuncture simply isn't for everyone. Some people may not be comfortable with the unusual nature of the treatment. Others may not have a reliable acupuncturist in their area. However, those who are willing to give acupuncture a try can experience many powerful benefits.

## Limit Alcohol

Alcohol is not a terrible thing. It is normal to enjoy a couple of drinks when hanging out with friends or out for a celebration. It makes you feel more confident and less worried because alcohol depresses your central nervous system. However, alcohol becomes an issue when used as an escape if you find yourself reaching for a drink when you feel upset or hopeless.

Alcohol temporarily increases the serotonin levels that your brain produces and then drops off as the alcohol leaves your body. Serotonin is a neurotransmitter in your brain that affects mood. When the alcohol wears off, you may feel even more anxious and depressed as your body recovers. Feelings of sickness and worry induced by being hungover can cause you to feel more unsettled. When you drink alcohol often, your brain rewires itself and tries to counteract the inhibition (being drunk) by building up your alcohol tolerance. What happens from there is that you can drink even more alcohol without feeling the effects, which will lead you to drink even more quantities.

## Limit Caffeine

If you are having trouble with anxiety, consider cutting down on your caffeine intake. Coffee, and sometimes strong teas, can cause your blood pressure to increase, along with your heart rate. If you are struggling with anxiety, you most likely already feel unsettled and jittery. Caffeine can increase these feelings. Also, caffeine blocks the neurotransmitter in your brain that makes you tired, so it can affect your sleep and keep you awake. Try substituting your morning cup of coffee for a cup of tea instead.

## Take Advantage of Sunshine

It is important to be outside. The sun provides vitamin D to your body, which is essential for your health. When the sun is shining bright on your shoulders or your face, you feel more active. It can help boost your mood, as the sun actually increases your levels of serotonin. Next time you are feeling down, take a step outside, face the sun, and close your eyes. Enjoy it and feel the warmth hugging your skin and let it rejuvenate you.

## Take a Deep Breath

When one feels anxious, sometimes the blood pressure levels go up; it is just natural stimuli to worry and experience nervousness. The person may experience increased or heavy breathing as the adrenaline levels go up. Whenever you are anxious, it is always wise to take a deep breath and systematically breathe in and out. Deep diaphragmatic breaths are a powerful technique to reduce anxiety levels; the process activates the body's relaxation response and eases the nerves. Deep breaths also help the body move from fight or flight mode to a controlled and calm nervous system.

Start by slowly breathing into a maximum count of four while filling the belly first, then the chest. Exercise your cardiac muscles by trying to hold your breath into a similar count of four gently. Slowly breathe out to a count of our and repeat this procedure several times until you feel your body relaxed.

## Accept That You Are Anxious

Anxiety is just a feeling like any other; let's say love, sympathy, and empathy; it only becomes a problem when it becomes a disorder, as I discussed earlier on. It is not a crime to be anxious, so do not judge yourself every time the feeling engulfs your system. By reminding yourself that anxiety is nothing more than a feeling and that you have the power to control it prepares you psychologically to confront the particular stimulus that causes your fear positively.

## Acknowledge That Your Brain is Playing Tricks on You

Thoughts are a powerful tool; they may influence your daily operations either positively or negatively. When an object, person, or situation causes high levels of fear to build up in you, your brain may, through the thoughts, emphasize the details to the point that you develop certain worries, fears, and phobias. During any panic attack, the brain quickly tries to get possible ways out of the situation, which is just in response to the cause of panic. Acting on an immediate impulse to your thoughts may not be the best decision; however, try out possible ways to calm your nerves and take time to debate on the range of remedies that your brain presents you. Once you can calm yourself and think of the many possible remedies, you have mentally overpowered your fear; anxiety leaves you helpless and always gives that feeling of defeat.

## Use a Calming Mental Picture or Visualization

Take stage fright. For example, fear may engulf you to the point that you may feel dizzy on stage. A mental picture distracts you and pulls part of your attention to other things that you best enjoy.

## Power of Positive Talk

Fear produces all sorts of negative thoughts that may be patent by negative chatter. Tell yourself positive affirming statements that build some little courage that will help you face the situation.

## Focus on the Moment

Anxiety knows no boundaries. It makes an individual focus on illogical occurrences of future events should the fear factor confront them. Every time you are anxious, do not bother about the future; rather, focus on what is happening to you at that particular time.

## Busy Yourself with Meaningful Activities

When the feeling of anxiety sets in, do not fret, an immediate relief can be achieved through focusing your attention on meaningful and goal-oriented activities. The anxiety interrupted a chain of activities that you were undertaking. If you were going shopping, still go and if you were planning to cook a nice meal still cook. The brain is always hungry for an idea; that's why we have numerous thoughts by the minute. Even when our bodies shut down, and we fall asleep, thoughts in the form of dreams still rampage our minds. The worst thing to do is just to sit down and do nothing when you are feeling anxious. Focusing on nothing means that you will focus on thoughts that will do you no good but intensify your worries.

## Self-Reward

Reward is positive reinforcement. Every time you overcome your fears, you can reward yourself with something that leaves a mark of assurance and emphasizes that inner voice that keeps telling you 'you can do it' every time you are anxious.

That was so much on achieving immediate anxiety relief; these steps can work for all anxiety disorders. You are advised to combine any three or more remedies any time you are reduced to an anxious fit.

## Meditation

There are so many types of meditation, and they are all aimed at fine-tuning your thoughts into positive energy that will reflect in most of your physical life. Meditation allows you ample time with yourself away from listening to what everyone is telling you about your condition. Every time you are anxious, take a deep breath and create a unique world of your own in your thoughts. Maintain a steady relationship with the air in the surroundings, the natural sounds, and your body's response to the stimuli introduced through meditation.

## Massage Your Worries Away

Massage has been used as a natural anxiety remedy for ages; it may be as simple as rubbing your neck gently, but whichever the case, you are massaging your way to calm nerves. The benefits of any massage therapy are many. Amongst them, stress relief, relaxation, lowers blood pressure, lowers tension build in the muscles, and improves deeper breathing. As the book unfolds, I will discuss therapeutic massage as a natural remedy for anxiety disorders. In this case, it will be much deeper and more precise.

## Having a Little Fun Never Killed Nobody

Laughing is a great relaxation technique and stress reliever. It increases lots of good feelings and serves to discharge tension. One major problem with people prone to anxiety is that they tend to take life so seriously that they appear to be melancholy all the time, and they eventually stop creating fun moments in their life. Fun and play are essential for the brain's proper functioning; it is a technique that stimulates the brain to come up with creative ideas rather than concentrating on unreasonable worries and fears. Within the fun and play, you may develop various ways to apply in situations when you are rendered anxious and helpless. Remember that rigidity limits you to a certain scope of ideas that will directly influence your take on the world.

## Tackle That Inner Voice (and Develop Your Positivity)

For many of us, the inner voice that provides the commentary to our every move isn't exactly kind. It can pull us up on our mistakes, criticize and whisper things that cut you right to the core. But if you can foster the support and encouragement of this inner voice, you can get through even the toughest times. Who better to love you than yourself, right?

What might come as a surprise is that you don't have to listen to this voice. You have the power to challenge it and make it dance to the beat of your drum, not its own. So next time it whispers hurtful things inside your ear, turn around and challenge it. Ask it what it is hoping to achieve and tell it you will only listen if it speaks to you with kindness.

Switch that negative inner voice to positive affirmations. Practice positive affirmations daily to calm your anxieties and transform your mindset into a positive and peaceful one. These affirmations can be anything that resonates with you.

Here are some simple yet powerful examples you can try:

- I feel cool, calm, and collected.
- Every part of the body is relaxed and light.
- With every breath, I let go of anxiety and feel calmer.
- I am confident that I will successfully tackle life's challenges.
- I feel at peace and can escape stress.
- I love myself deeply and unconditionally.
- All is well in my world and I am safe.
- I look forward to my future with hope and happiness.
- I can overcome my fears and live life courageously.

## Taking Care of Your Body

There is a strong relationship between mind, emotion, and body. It will be easier to relax if you know that you are taking care of your body. Try to develop healthy eating and fitness eating habits. Exercise and a clean diet can do wonders for your anxiety.

Also, try to sleep well and on time. If you have a healthy routine, you will have more energy to face and handle life's ups and downs. Make wise food choices, develop a good sleeping habit, and exercise regularly. It sounds far too simple, but this has been one of the biggest factors in overcoming anxiety.

## Talk About Your Problems with Other People

It helps if you have a trusted friend or relative who is willing to listen to your worries. Trying to contain your feelings can be very challenging. It will just allow your panic to snowball. When a person is willing to listen to your problems and vulnerabilities, you will be a bit more at ease and realize that you are not alone, and secondly, things aren't as bad as they seem.

Do not always expect that the other person will be able to comfort you completely. It is highly unlikely that the other person will be able to erase all your worries. However, talking about worries will prevent them from becoming bigger and bigger. It will prevent you from snapping in an unexpected situation. Talking about your problems will prevent you from exploding and may assist you in maintaining perspective.

## Try Connecting with Nature

There is something about the harmony of nature which is incredibly calming and relaxing. Allow yourself to be comforted by the beauty of the universe. Find solace in parks or gardens. Choose a place that will make you feel safe and grounded. If you want, you can even ask a friend to accompany you as you enjoy nature's wonders. I love sitting on a bench in a park on a quiet Sunday morning and just watching the world go by. I may choose to read a book or simply sit and contemplate life and my surroundings. This has an amazing calming effect and allows me to ensure I see the world in all its beauty and splendor.

You can also engage in a hobby involving nature. Gardening or mountain climbing is a good way to improve your relationship with the wonders around you. You'll be surprised by what a little sunshine can do in your life. You will feel lighter, better, and maybe even happier.

## Try to Be Grateful

To be honest, there are a million and one ways that things can go wrong in every moment. Your situation could be much worse than it is. Try to focus on the good things that are happening in your life. Look for things that you can be grateful for. Do you have a roof above your head? Are there people in your life that make you smile? If you focus on the good things that happen in your life, you will likely feel less anxious about what the future holds.

## Try to Learn To Calm Yourself Down

People sometimes become slaves to their feelings. If you are anxious, you need to learn how to find your peace of mind. Find your own "calm" place. That means knowing how to take charge when it seems like your emotions are taking over. There are many various ways to calm yourself down.

## Learn to Keep Yourself Busy

If you are an anxiety sufferer, you will likely spend your free time worrying about unimportant things. Try to minimize your idle time so that you won't spend too much time worrying about things that don't matter. It is best to try and get a hobby to fill up your free time. Find something that interests you. It is a good idea to get into art or sports. Besides keeping you busy, it will also help you use up your energy, so you won't have excess energy to worry about silly things that don't matter.

## Practice Mindfulness

At times, we become so caught up in our minds that we forget to be present in the world around us and miss out on much of the beauty of life. Instead, we see the looming deadlines and stressful obligations instead of breathing in the joy. So slow down, open your eyes to the things that are right there around you and find things to be grateful for.

## Meditation

Mediation is fast becoming one of the most popular self-help and wellness techniques of all time and is no longer a preserve of the 'green' crowds. Regularly practicing will help lower your heart rate, rebalance your hormones, help you to become more mindful, and stop your stress response right in its tracks. Why not give it a try; challenge yourself to meditate for just 30 days and see how much better you will feel.

Here's a great exercise to get started with:

- Sit down somewhere comfortable where you will not be disturbed for the duration of your practice and set your timer for an allotted time. Just 10 minutes can be effective, especially when you begin.
- Adopt a comfortable position with your feet flat on the floor and your hands resting lightly in your lap.
- Now focus your attention on the movement of your breath as it enters and leaves your body. Do not attempt to change it. Simply, observe.
- Begin to count your inhalations starting at one, up to a count of 10, and then repeat for as long as you wish.
- Next, count your exhalations up to a count of 10 again until you feel the desire to switch to a different technique.
- While you are focusing your attention in this manner, try to relax your mind as much as you can. You don't need to try to make your mind go blank, but instead simply acknowledge your thoughts and allow them to float past you. That might be difficult for you at first, but you will improve as you continue to practice.
- After the allotted period, simply open your eyes and gently return to reality.

## Use Positive Visualization

Positive visualization is the super-effective technique that most top athletes, business people, and high achievers utilize to get them the results they want. By picturing the outcome that you dream of, you are more able to move forwards towards your biggest goals, overcome any obstacles that might come across your path, and also fall in love with the journey itself.

## Work with a Therapist

Don't be afraid of working with a therapist if your stress or anxiety is severely interfering with your quality of life. Holistic help is only taking the edge off the problem. Therapists are experienced individuals who have been trained to understand what you are going through and can provide that unconditional support to prevent you from descending into more serious anxiety disorders, depression, or stress-related disorders.

## Tai Chi and Yoga

Being another stress and anxiety-killing activity, yoga involves stretching and deep breathing. Variations of yoga poses bring awareness to muscles that you may not use daily. I carry my stress in my neck and my shoulders. Yoga helps stretch those muscles and relieve the tension from my body. Another important aspect of yoga is the inward focus as well. Focusing on your breath is also an important yoga practice. That ensures that you are delivering enough oxygen to your muscles as you stretch them. Yoga and meditation can be used together for the ultimate anxiety-relieving experience.

Both yoga and tai chi are also effective relaxation exercises. Yoga can improve the body's relaxation response in day-to-day life. These exercises are slow-paced and not at all strenuous, making them a good fit for people of all ages.

Those who are unfamiliar with yoga and tai chi may want to begin by taking a class. Some moves are hard to imitate without seeing them in motion. Video footage is also an option.

From deep breathing to full body stretches, relaxation exercises can provide long-term and short-term relationships. Once these techniques become a regular part of a person's life, they'll find that they feel far calmer and experience far less anxiety.

Relaxation exercises can provide people with a great deal of control over their anxiety symptoms. When regularly practiced, these techniques can help people to experience fewer symptoms and far fewer panic attacks. They're something anxiety sufferers should familiarize themselves with.

## Psychotherapy

Psychotherapy is also called talk therapy, and it has been seen as effective in helping people suffering from anxiety disorders in coping with their anxiety. Psychotherapy always needs to be given at the specific level of a person's anxiety to work effectively. Engaging in psychotherapy may be difficult for the person suffering from an anxiety disorder. He finds it extremely difficult to discuss his anxiety-provoking triggers and situations and feels extremely uncomfortable at first when discussed about facing his fears.

## Cognitive Behavioral Therapy (CBT)

CBT is a very popular type of modern psychotherapy that has helped people deal with their anxiety disorders. Through CBT, a person's way of thinking, behavior, and how he reacts to situations that cause anxiety or make him fearful can be altered productively. CBT helps people learn and apply social skills in their lives, which is the core of social Anxiety.

# DR. SEBI'S RECCOMENDED LIFESTYLE CHANGES TO IMPROVE YOUR CANCER CARE

People with cancer will experience a variety of symptoms, but there is one factor that is common no matter what illness they have: the anxiety that comes with not knowing what the future holds. As a result, many cancer patients find comfort in the doctor's assurance that all will be okay. However, this emotional support can sometimes be false and misguided. If you want to live your life, rather than simply focus on surviving it, here are Dr. Sebi's recommendations for how to improve your care for cancer without breaking the bank or changing your lifestyle too drastically.

## ACCEPT PRACTICAL AND EMOTIONAL SUPPORT

*Seek out low-cost cancer treatment centers*

If you want to live your life instead of struggling to survive it, then find a clinic that's willing to work with you financially. Cancer treatment can be very expensive, especially when the patient needs special medication not covered by insurance; therefore, if you need help lowering costs, don't hesitate to ask for it. A clinic that works with alternative medicine and has a strong focus on nutrition will be able to help you save money on your treatment.

*Talk to your doctor about supplements and other alternative treatments*

There are many other ways to help with cancer without going under the knife; talk to your doctor if appropriate. There are natural supplements that can have a positive effect on some cancers, while others will be helped by specific foods or even vitamins and minerals used in cleanses. Some people will be able to reduce the symptoms of cancer by drinking fresh juices and even wine when treating themselves with alternative treatments.

Consider practicing a more natural lifestyle.

There are certain things that people should avoid doing while they are having treatment, but on the whole, living in an insanitary environment can have a detrimental effect on someone with cancer.

*Learn how to use your own body's healing powers*

If you want to really treat your cancer naturally, then start learning about the ways that you can use your own body's healing powers to make yourself better. The more you know about this, the less dependent on outside sources you will be for treatment. The journey of health is a lifelong one, and there is no reason why someone with cancer can't get on that road early by eating well, exercising and staying in good spirits throughout treatment.

# MANAGE STRESS

Stress is a common, yet harmful, part of life. When you are stressed, your immune system decreases and leaves your body more vulnerable to side effects from chemo treatments or radiation therapy. Stress also can lead to depression and anxiety.

Stress can take many forms in terms of your cancer treatment. It may be the fear of dealing with a life-threatening illness. There also can be stresses related to physical symptoms, such as hair loss from chemo or fatigue from radiation therapy. The emotional burden of being diagnosed with cancer, and the financial stress from mounting bills also are significant sources of stress for cancer patients. In addition, you also may feel stressed about missing work because of treatments or about taking time off for doctor appointments.

You can control many sources of stress in your life. These include how you choose to spend your time, how you deal with stressors, and how you deal with the new challenges of cancer treatment. By learning the habits that help you cope effectively with stress in your life, you can take action steps to face life's challenges more successfully.

Here are some ways to help reduce the impact of stress upon your cancer care:

Make time for yourself. Cancer treatment leaves you tired and may disrupt family and work activities. You also may feel a sense of isolation as other people become less accessible during treatment or recovery. Making time for yourself helps give you balance in your daily life and helps motivate you through stressful periods of cancer treatment. Try to schedule activities that bring you pleasure, such as taking walks, reading, gardening and going to the movies.

Find relaxation activities. This could be a hobby or a hobby activity that relaxes you. It also can include getting massages or scheduling a massage for yourself. Relaxation is important to help reduce the stress of cancer treatment. Massages are especially effective at reducing stress because they are physically therapeutic and emotionally relaxing.

Manage stressors in your life. Cancer treatment causes so many stressors in your life that it is difficult to cope effectively with them all. You cannot change some stressors, but you can manage others. Reduce stressors by avoiding people who make you feel stressed, learning to control your anger, and avoiding situations that cause emotional stress.

For example, if a loved one is pressuring you to do something against your own wishes, it is time to set a limit. Tell that person directly how his or her behavior affects you and how he or she can change their behavior so that it does not cause stress for you.

Handling anger is another way to reduce the stress of cancer treatment. Learning how to manage your anger when you are angry helps reduce the long-term effects of anger on your health.

Talk about the stress of cancer treatment. Discuss your feelings and thoughts with a friend or family member you trust. Cancer is a difficult time for every family, and talking with someone who understands may help reduce stress.

Get support from others. Learn what sources of support are available if you need help managing your stress levels during cancer treatment. You may be able to connect with peers through support groups sponsored by hospitals or other cancer organizations.

## GET ENOUGH SLEEP

As many as 70 million Americans suffer from insomnia and sleep disorders, the effects of which can include depression, heart disease, and other health related issues. One common sleep disorder is obstructive sleep apnea (OSA) which affects up to 20% of Americans. In fact, many people with OSA are undiagnosed.

It's important for cancer patients to get enough quality sleep in order to tackle their recovery journey with a renewed vigor and spirit. Not only does sleep help cancer patients heal, but it also has a direct effect on the effectiveness of chemotherapy and other cancer medications. Cancer patients should aim for 8 hours of sleep per night to get the full benefits of nighttime rest.

## EXERCISE REGULARLY

Exercise daily even if it's difficult initially

It is important to get some form of exercise throughout your life; no matter what, you have to keep moving so that all those toxins aren't sucked up through your skin into your bloodstream. This will help you lose some weight and make you feel better about your health. If going to the gym is out of the question, then perform daily exercises in your home or a park.

## EAT WELL

Eat organic foods and drink clean water daily

While you may be eating healthy foods at home and drinking clean water from the tap, you need to make sure that your food comes from the supermarket. There is a vast difference between a food that was grown in your own back yard and one that has been transported around the country while being treated with chemicals. Canned goods are also quite a waste of money when they can be replaced at home with fresh fruits and vegetables.

## AVOID ENVIRONMENTAL TOXINS

Replace chemical-based products with natural and organic ones.

Chemicals are present in most synthetic products, including cosmetics and personal care items. Avoid using these as much as possible and replace them with natural, organic versions instead. There is something particularly upsetting about seeing a person with cancer slather themselves in chemical-based hair dye or makeup; it may not be the best choice for cancer patients to visit salons unless they are specifically geared toward these kinds of treatments. It is important to avoid using products that contain chemicals at all costs, but if you must use them then make sure that they are certified organics so that you can minimize the effects they will have on your body in the long run.

## AVOID SMOKING AND DRINKING ALCOHOL

While it may seem like common sense, it bears repeating that smoking and drinking alcohol should be avoided as much as possible while undergoing cancer treatment. Smoking contains dangerous chemicals that will only further complicate the condition of a cancer patient. Alcohol is also known to cause aggressive cancers, so the less contact a person has with it, the better. You don't have to go on a full detox after being diagnosed with cancer; simply try avoiding these two unhealthy habits as much as possible for now to improve your chances of living with this illness without any adverse effects.

## ACIDIC BODY, MUCUS BUILD-UP AND DISEASES

D r. Sebi said that If there is extra mucus in the bronchial channels, the disease is known as bronchitis; if the lungs are affected, the disease will be pneumonia; if it affects the pancreatic duct, then it is diabetes, and if it affects the joints, it's arthritis."

According to Dr. Sebi, "Mucus is the source of any illness," the easiest way to eliminate phlegm is by consuming the right foods.

### What is Mucus?

Mucus appears to be an unpleasant material secreted by our bodies, but it is created to defend us from bacteria and other pathogens in reality.

Mucus is an aqueous substance formed by mucosal surfaces that line some hollow organs linked to the eternal body, such as the gastrointestinal canal, airway tract, sinuses, and genital organs.

### How is mucus created in the body?

If a foreign object disturbs or invades a membrane liner, inflammation starts. Inflammation is thus a battle between the body's protective cells and invasive pathogens. The immune cells activate the production of a chemical named histamine during inflammation. This chemical allows the blood vessels dilation enabling more blood to circulate to the area of inflammation. It not only encourages more WBC (white blood cells) to be released at the area, it also enables the mucous membranes to release more mucus.

### The Mucus Function

The pathogen-fighting cells produce mucus as one of their arms. In exchange, the captured bacteria are killed by the body's protective cells.

This fluid includes antibodies and enzymes that digest harmful substances we are exposed to. Although the body can mean well as it releases mucus, persistent secretion can indicate that the body is in a condition of chronic inflammation, which raises the risk of cancer, cardiac disease, and diabetes, among other health problems.

### Impact of excess mucus in the body

Symptoms and signs of abnormal mucosa:

Mucus formation has several uses, even though you are healthy. It covers the tissues that line the throat, lungs, nose, sinus, and nasal passages and prevents them from drying up. Mucus produces enzymes and antibodies that destroy or neutralize toxic bacteria in the air. Assume about it as a line of protection that will protect you from getting ill.

If everything functions exactly as intended, you are not even going to notice the mucus. But the color of mucus changes if there is an infection. You can produce more

mucus than normal if you smoke cigarettes or are allergic to a stimulant in the air. If you begin to make so much visible mucus, it could suggest that you have allergies and that your body is getting rid of allergens like dust or pollen. If you have a cold, bronchitis, or sinus infection, your mucus can turn greenish, yellow, or beige. The explanation for that? Once you get an infection, the body generates additional white blood cells and distributes them to your respiratory tract to combat it. These white blood cells produce a neutrophil compound, which may add a greenish or yellow hue to the mucus. Mucus can often tend to be green when thickened.

This is also an indication that blood is present in the mucus, which is usually the product of inflammation or when the tissue lining of the nasal passages drying out, caused by constant scratching, brushing or blowing the nose.

There isn't much to think about, a tiny bit of blood on the mucus. But if you have heavy bleeding, speak to the doctor. It may be a symptom of a dangerous illness, such as pneumonia, bronchitis, or even cancer. Phlegm, a form of mucus, is formed by the respiratory system and lungs. It is a symbol of irritation and inflammation. (The nose creates the mucus.) You might have heard the word sputum—this is phlegm that you eject by coughing.

If extra mucus is the only symptom, it is not usually anything to think about.

## *Factors and Predisposing Causes of Mucus*

When you are ill, the body does not necessarily generate more mucus, while it may seem like that. What you see is more definitely a difference in its consistency. Your mucus can get stickier or thicker. It will build up in the throat and lungs at elevated amounts, contributing to troubled breathing and swallowing.

As a consequence of this buildup, you can feel a postnasal trickle. This happens as extra mucus drips in the throat from the back of the nose. It also contributes to coughing.

You could have dry mucous membranes if you have excessive mucus buildup. And it may be due to the following reasons

Dry indoor surroundings (due to air-conditioning or heat)

Not consuming an adequate amount of water or other liquids

Drinking liquids such as coffee, tea, or beer, which can contribute to dehydration.

Taking some particular medicines

Smoking

Increased mucus can be a complication of COPD (chronic obstructive pulmonary disease), bronchitis, cystic fibrosis. Or bronchiectasis, or

Primary ciliary dyskinesia

Primary ciliary dyskinesia is normally an autosomal recessive syndrome. A ciliary impairment inhibits mucosal clearance from the lungs, middle ears, and nasal cavity Bacteria and other mucosal irritants contribute to regular respiratory infections.

Affected patients also suffer persistent sinus, lung, and middle ear infections, persistent coughing, excessive mucus, and hearing problems. Recurrent respiratory infections may contribute to permanent scarring and dilation of the bronchi (bronchiectasis) and serious lung harm.

Cystic Fibrosis:

Cystic fibroid mucus in people becomes dehydrated and becoming so dense and moist that cilia cannot push mucus from their lungs. As a consequence, the mucus blocks the airways, rendering it impossible to breathe. Since mucus in people with Cystic Fibrosis r is often unusual in some respects, it is less likely to destroy germs like the mucus in healthy people, making a favorable environment for infections.

## Ulcerative Colitis

The mucus surface of the large intestine produces mucus. Mucus is often formed by other organs and systems, like the lungs, where it captures foreign particles breathed in. In the digestive tract, mucus covers the inside of the padding, which, since it is oily, facilitates the feces' movement.

Having to pass mucus in the feces is not dangerous on its own since it is a natural part of the stool, although so much may also be a symptom of an illness or condition that could need medication. If the mucus coating is shed too much, it might cause the colon more vulnerable to bacteria.

Ulcerative Colitis is one such factor that contributes to noticeable mucus, the stool in the mucus layer of the large intestine (colon). In ulcerative Colitis, it gets inflamed and produces small sores or ulcers. Such ulcers bleed and can also cause mucus and mucus. The mucus can be thick enough to be noticed when it passes along with the feces

## Dr. Sebi's Cure to Rid Excess Mucus

Understanding the alkalinity-acidity equilibrium is an integral aspect of anyone's health toolkit. Dr. Sebi brought a refreshing insight into what living an alkaline life is like. Fight the symptoms of increased acidity and learn more about alkaline things to minimize extra mucus in the body.

What is the equilibrium between acid and alkaline? The pH range tests our body systems acidic and alkalinity, and the scale is 0-14. The pH is 7.0. More alkaline has stronger pH (greater than 7), whereas the lower pH is acidic (less than 7). Our bodies must be mildly alkaline for excellent wellbeing. Our immunity is strongly connected to the way our food is alkaline. An excessively acidic diet ultimately causes our bodies to become disease-prone, and The nervous tract, the liver, and the kidneys all start to suffer. It leads to several problems, including asthma, allergies, inflammation, constipation, arthritis, and other bowel problems. It is really difficult for the body to build an equilibrium.

And should we be worried about the "alkalization" of our bodies daily? Your body is actively attempting to get you around to a more alkaline condition while you are depressed, making bad lifestyle decisions, or are subjected to a toxic atmosphere. The body begins pulling from the muscles, teeth, and organs to neutralize acid minerals such as magnesium and calcium. Unprocessed plant food is extremely alkaline, which means that it cleanses the blood, oxidizes the body, and keeps your body's cells in top shape! It provides you with energy, clears your skin, and reduces your body's inflammation.

Where are we supposed to begin? You are welcome to start the day with regular citrus waters and drink a green veggies juice, and at any meal, you should load more than half your dish with vegetables. Balance overly acidic items such as sugar, milk, beef, alcohol, and caffeine by regularly stocking on salads, organic vegetables, berries, and alkaline water. Approximately 80/20: Allow 80% alkaline and 20% acidic foods in your diet.

Follow these easy guidelines to alkalize the body daily:

Drink more water

The adequate consumption of water benefits all systems of the body and removes excess toxins. Drink half of your body weight per day in ounces to maintain your body systems. For example, drink 65 oz. of water every day if you are 130 pounds. Get a flask of water and fill it with water (filtered); continuously drinking in plastic glasses causes hormones to become damaging. Add lemon for additional improvement in alkalinity! Not just alkalizing lemon water, but it often provides large quantities of vitamin C and digestive aids.

Have tea instead of coffee.

Green tea has strong alkaline content. Check jasmine, matcha, or Sencha - or change to a less refined coffee that is less acidic such as bulletproofs or 'no acid' labels.

Both materials used by the dental office should be ecologically friendly.

Instead of sugar, use coconut sugar stevia or limited quantities of honey. Sugar is by far the most acidic item of our everyday lives, and it comes out everywhere. Try to balance as often as possible by incorporating different sweeteners.

Get a higher consumption of green vegetables

Have salads and/greens in your diet. Load up every meal with leafy greens. Add up a tablespoon with green powder, or purchase liquid chlorophyll and add chlorophyll to your drink once a day. Greens are rich in oxygen and heavily alkaline. Drink as much as possible organic green vegetable juices. Again, greens have large chlorophyll levels that contain more oxygen and oxygen Equals to alkalinity.

Move more

Exercise in building more oxygen and energy in the body and prevent stagnation. Dance, walk, do yoga, play, and enjoy yourself with your children! Exercise frequently contributes to stress relief. Whenever you may, be on your feet and walk about; whenever you move your body, you raise the concentration of oxygen in your blood, increasing the alkalinity in your blood.

Reduce the level of the stress

Meditate as much as possible, do deep meditation, perform yoga, go out in nature, try the earthing, and have a good sleep. Go for a stroll after dinner – anything that helps you feel centered, sip tea, daydream. Cellular acidity is generated by stress. Try to stabilize yourself by making routines to help your body and mind feel good and peaceful.

## Essential Tools & Instruments

You cannot just get up and run towards the wilderness to start foraging. You have to be well trained and well equipped before you do that.

It's not like you have to go out there and start searching for different plants that you can eat, and on finding one, you can pull the whole plant out of the earth. You have to be careful about foraging.

You should get trained first to know about the essential tools you need for foraging in the wilderness.

The Forager's Toolkit

First of all, you would need a forager's toolkit. What should that toolkit contain? Let's have a look:

Transport Containers

This is the most important thing that a forager must have when he is foraging. If you have collected enough plants and herbs from foraging, you need containers to carry them home.

These containers can be in different shapes and sizes depending on your foraging loot. There are many different plants and herbs that you forage, so depending on their types and the season that you would be foraging in, keep the following containers in your forager's toolkit always,

Plastic Bags:

If you are going to forage plants and herbs in large quantities, plastic shopping bags will prove to be helpful. You can collect mallow, purslane, will mustard, etc., in plastic bags. Also, if you are planning on foraging bigger fruits and nuts like apples, walnuts, or lemons, plastic bags can come in handy.

Sandwich Bags:

When you are foraging for tiny things like different kinds of seeds and pine nuts etc., you should have sandwich bags in your toolkit. These bags are good for collecting things is too little for plastic shopping bags.

Freezer Bags:

If you find larger plants like plantain plants or sumac, you can keep them in freezer bags. They should be in your toolkit when you are foraging for things too big for sandwich bags, but if you put them in plastic shopping bags, you can lose them through the small holes.

Covered Containers:

Covered containers like Tupperware are also an essential part of your forager's toolkit. They can be used when you are foraging things that would be crushed in different kinds of bags.

The things next to the bags would crush the items in the plastic bag, so it is better to use Tupperware of covered containers for such delicate things.

Fruits like grapes, apricots, different kinds of berries, etc., can be crushed easily. So, instead of putting them in a plastic bag, you should always have a covered container with you.

Tupperware is also good for putting flowers and some thorny foods like milk thistle and prickly pear, which can tear the sides of the bags.

Picking Aids

Like I have mentioned before, you cannot just go on and pull out the whole plant or a young tree by your hand when you are foraging. You have to have some tools to save the plants and herbs and save your hands if you find something prickly or thorny.

The following picking aids are essential for your forager's toolkit,

A pair of scissors:

You will find all sorts of plants when you go on foraging in the wilderness. Some plants, you will be able to pick easily with just a slight movement of your fingers without any real hard work, and there are some plants that you will have to twist once or twice and bend back and forth with your hands until the stem breaks, and you get the plant you want.

But you will also find some plants in the wilderness that would not only be difficult to break with your bare hands, but also, they will resist your efforts to breaking them. In doing so, if you keep pushing and pulling, the whole plant might get damaged, or the whole plant might break when all you want to pick was a fruit.

Also, you cannot pick plants that are prickly and thorny with your bare hands. To avoid trouble in such cases, you should always have a pair of scissors in your forager's toolkit.

You can cut the plant from the lower part of the stem instead of damaging the roots by pulling out the whole plant. This way, the plant would be safe, and it would keep growing.

Your fingers will also remain unscathed if you are using a pair of scissors to cut plants like stinging nettles.

Gardening Gloves:

Gardening gloves offer a lot of protection to your hand when you are foraging. They keep your hands from getting cut by thorny plants like stinging nettles. It is safe to use gardening gloves anyway when you are foraging.

Hard Plastic or Cardboard Mitts:

Gardening gloves are good for keeping your hands safe from thorns and spikes of different plants, but sometimes, even gardening gloves cannot give you enough protection. Some thorns would tear through your gardening gloves and cut your hands.

Gardening gloves keep the thorns and spikes embedded in your gloves that would cut your hands the next time you wear them to foraging, even if you are not anywhere near a spiky plant.

These spikes don't come out even when you wash the gloves. After you wear your gardening gloves while handling some plants with thorns, you would have to throw them out. You cannot use them the next time.

So, it is a good idea to make your gloves from a material that the thorns cannot cut through.

You can use plastic soda bottles. Cut one end of the bottle and use the other end of the plastic soda bottle as a "mitt." You can hold the bottle from outside and cup the prickly pear in the hole you cut in the bottle.

You can then squeeze the bottle shut to trap the prickly pear inside. Twist the bottle, and you would get the prickly pear without damaging your hands.

You should also keep the cardboard in your forager's toolkit to pick up things like prickly pears to milk thistle. Wrap the plant with a cardboard piece and then grab the cardboard to pick the thorny plant.

Long Sticks:

When you are foraging, you will find various fruits on your journey. If you find fruit on an unreachable branch of a tall tree, what would you do? For this, you should always have a long stick to shake the tree's branches so that the fruits and nuts can fall and you can forage them.

Mini Hand Trowel:

You have learned in this book about some plants whose roots can be eaten too. For this purpose, a mini hand trowel is an essential tool that should always be in your forager's toolkit.

You can dig with your hands too, but a mini trowel would get the job done faster than your bare hands, and it would be a lot less messy.

For a beginner, the forager mentioned above's tools are good for a start. All the tools mentioned above are essential for foraging.

## Wildcrafting

Wildcrafting is probably the most ancient activity men have ever done. It consists of harvesting plants from the wild for food or medicinal purposes. When done sustainably, this is a win-win for both men and plants: men can receive food or medicinal herbs from nature, and in exchange, they take care of the surrounding environment by taking only what is necessary, replanting plants and seeds, removing dead branches to help the plant grow faster and more robust. There are techniques and gathering methods that allow the plant and the surrounding environment to benefit from the harvesting. This is important to minimize the impact we have on our planet and ensure that we have access to nature's benefits for many generations to come.

## Planting and Harvesting

Wildcrafting is the practice of foraging for useful plants from their natural, wild habitat for edible or medicinal purposes. These plants are gathered to be used as food and medicine from their natural habitat. It is for medicinal herbs and is one of the most rewarding things. Nowadays, wildcrafters gather and dry various botanicals to be shipped to buyers. They search the woods and fields to find varieties of plants, both rare and common. However, certain parts of each plant are valuable such as leaves, bark and stems and they are collected as herbs.

## Drying and Storing Herbs

It is a good idea to dry and store your herbs. This will control the lifespan of all herbs. Drying is a good option for most types of herbs- it preserves the flavor, color, and texture of the original herb. The type of herb dictates if drying or freezing is better for storage purposes.

Follow these steps to get started:

1. Gather clean materials such as paper towels, a wire rack, clean sheets or cloths, and large containers with lids.
2. Cut your herbs into small pieces that will fit in a bowl or jar with room at the top for air circulation. Place these in a single layer on two layers of paper towels on top of a wire rack over a paper towel-lined tray.
3. Dry the herbs at room temperature or remove from the paper towels to air dry. It is important that the herbs are not exposed to direct sunlight for an extended period of time, as this can make them prone to molding. If it is not possible to dry them in an airtight container, use an oven-proof one with a tight-fitting lid for overnight drying. You can't use plastic containers or plastic bags for this process because they do not retain the moisture of the herb dried.
4. Once the herbs are finished, store them in a cool place away from sunlight and ready-to-eat temperatures for later use.

There are two choices for storing your dried herbs. The first option is to store them in airtight containers. This is recommended if the herbs will be used often, or if they are needed after a short period of time.

The second option is to freeze them. This keeps them fresh for up to 6 months, and only needs the transfer of the frozen herb to one container for storage (this makes it easier when using them in various recipes). Some herbs that do not freeze well are cilantro, basil, mint, and parsley.

To use frozen herbs: allow them to thaw out at room temperature or by microwaving for about 10 seconds. They do not need to be washed prior to use. Once the herbs are completely melted, use as you would fresh herbs.

Another alternative is to make herb powders (such as rosemary, thyme, and bay leaf). This is done by grinding dried herbs in a blender or food processor with another food item such as sugar or salt.

This process makes them easier for cooking and storage purposes.

The larger the herb pieces that are dried, the longer they will last in storage. It is also a good idea to store dried herbs and spice mixes in airtight containers and sealable bags so they do not lose their flavor or aroma before they are used up.

Rosemary –The leaves of this plant are often used as a flavoring and to flavor breads and pastries.

Cilantro – This herb is used extensively in Mexican and South Asian foods, but it can also be found in other cuisines such as Italian and Mediterranean. It is mostly grown in Mexico, but can also be found growing wild in some areas of America such as California.

Basil – Although basil has many uses throughout the culinary world, it is most commonly used as an aromatic spice that provides a distinct flavor to certain dishes such as pesto. Basil is the national herb of Italy.

Bay – This herb is used to flavor Mexican foods such as beans and beef. It is also a favorite among chefs for its distinct aroma and flavor. It can be found growing wild in certain areas of the United States such as California.

Mint – This herb is used to flavor breads, pastries, and sauces throughout the world. It is often used as a substitute for peppermint oil in many types of candy.

Thyme, Lemon Balm & Rosemary -These herbs are also some popular spices that can be found in some cuisines around the world. Thyme is mostly grown in Italy while lemon balm and rosemary are grown throughout Europe and North America.

Parsley -Parsley is more of a root than an herb. It is used to flavor soups, stews, and sauces throughout the world.

Chives – These tiny green onion-like leaves are known for their distinctive flavor and smell. They are often used in dishes like soups, salads, and side dishes.

Basil (fresh) - This type of basil is most commonly found in Italian cuisine. It has a distinct flavor that enhances the flavor of many different kinds of foods. It is also known for its ability to lower blood pressure, improve circulation, and lower cholesterol levels due to its high vitamin C content.

## Foraging

Foraging and harvesting are a way of life for the Native Americans in the Pacific Northwest. They committed to it because they understood that they had to provide for themselves while respecting nature.

Foraging and harvesting are two of the mainstays of Native American life. Native Americans would carefully choose which plants they collected, identifying them by taste, smell, and sight. They would then prepare them in dishes with other ingredients like wild game or fish. Here are some tips for identifying plants that can help you start your journey and see how the natives lived!

## Foraging

It is a skill that all Native Americans need to know. Foraging can be dangerous, so you should always have a full stomach before going out foraging. You should be with someone that knows what to do if you get lost or something terrible happens.

Foraging was also one way for the Native American people to learn about their environment and become more spiritually connected. For example, the plants in the area were used for almost every need. The Native Americans used plants like cedar and spruce for clothing and blankets and made baskets, mats, and clothing. They used bark from trees to build shelters or to cover themselves at night. The berries were used for food and medicine; they had properties that kept animals away or killed parasites. Even in the Pacific Northwest, it was essential for their survival to know how to use what nature gave them.

## Reaping

It is among the most essential and sacred tasks of Native Americans to put in the necessary time and effort to harvest plants for food, medicine, and other purposes. Spring through fall is some of the best times of the year for gathering many types of plants. People of all ages participate in harvesting plants, and it is often a family project.

The plants harvested by Native Americans include many kinds of berries, such as pokeberry and blackberry. Native Americans also harvest grasses such as Indian ricegrass for their food value. The juice from the stalks of Indian ricegrass can be squeezed into a cup or bowl to make a nutritious drink.

The crinkle-seed plant roots can be dug up, cleaned, and eaten raw or dried and used as flour for making bread or cakes. Nettles can be picked and cooked with other greens as a tasty side dish.

It is essential to acknowledge this evidence of the people's ability to adapt, contributing to their survival for so many years. It allows us as a society to make a connection with the Native Americans and what they have had to endure.

Like many cultures worldwide, the Native Americans relied on seasonal harvests of wild foods such as berries, roots, and furs. They also hunted certain animals during certain times of the year, like salmon, when they swam upstream towards their spawning grounds. To catch fish, they used multiple methods like setting nets, spearing, or using hooks. The Pacific Northwest Native Americans often harvested salmon to provide for their families or trade with others. They would preserve the fish by smoking, drying, or making it into a dried food good called pemmican.

## ALKALINE HERBAL REMEDIES FOR COMMON AILMENTS

### Abscess and Gingivitis

#### HERBAL MOUTHWASH

This powerful antimicrobial mouthwash can help fight bacteria that lead to gingivitis, as well as treat sores in the mouth. This can be created with a combination of sage and pau d' arco. Start by boiling two cups of water on the stove. Add one teaspoon of sage and one teaspoon of pau d' arco bark. Let this simmer for ten to fifteen minutes or until the liquid is reduced by half. Remove it from heat and set it aside to cool a little. When it is still warm, add one teaspoon of sea salt or Himalayan salt. Blend until the salt has dissolved into the mixture. Let this cool completely and strain everything out into a glass jar for storage. Store this in the refrigerator between uses. For oral care or for treating oral sores, gargle one teaspoon of this mouthwash for two minutes. Repeat this up to three times daily until the sore has healed. For oral maintenance, gargle once daily.

#### SKIN ABSCESS FIGHTING TEA

Skin abscesses are often the result of a bacterial infection under several layers of the skin's surface. Oftentimes, these happen in areas of the body that are bothered by constant pressure or clothing that rubs the area a lot. Pay attention to your body and any areas that feel sore. If you feel a skin abscess in common areas like around the waist (where pants rub) or the bra line (for women it is very common to get abscesses in this area because undergarments rub it) take action right away to treat it. If an abscess is left untreated, it can develop into a much more severe infection and require lancing, which can be very painful. You can take care of an abscess without resulting to a painful procedure with a tea made form yellow dock root. Yellow dock roots are very detoxifying and purifying. They can cleanse the body from the inside out. Infuse one teaspoon of dried yellow dock root into one cup of hot water. Let this infuse for up to ten minutes. Drink up to three cups daily to promote the elimination of bacteria from the abscess. Use this treatment in conjunction with the next treatment for abscesses.

## TOPICAL WASH FOR ABSCESSES AND GINGIVITIS

Take on an abscess of any form of bacteria with an antimicrobial and antibiotic topical wash made from yarrow and Cordoncillo negro leaves. Both of these herbs help to kill bacteria and treat skin issues that result from bacterial infections. Make a strong decoction with these to by boiling three cups of water on the stove and adding one tablespoon each of dried yarrow and Cordoncillo negro leaves. Reduce the heat to simmer and let this infuse for up to twenty minutes. Try to get the liquid to reduce by at least half. Allow the liquid to cool. Strain it out when it has cooled and store it in a glass jar. Refrigerate it between uses. In the refrigerator, it should last up to three weeks. You can use this in two ways. The first way is to use it for compresses on the affected area. This is very helpful for treating an abscess. Soak a small clean rag in the liquid and apply it to the area as needed until the abscess is gone. For gingivitis, simply gargle the liquid for one minute up to three times daily, depending on the severity of the case.

## Acne

### SKIN TONER

For a gentle yet effective skin toner that works under the surface of the skin to kill the bacteria that lead to acne, try a skin toner made with chamomile and sage. Sage kills bacteria that lead to acne and chamomile reduces redness and evens out skin tone. Together, these two herbs are the perfect combination for creating a clear complexion. Start by boiling one teaspoon each of sage and chamomile in two cups of water. Reduce heat and let this simmer until the liquid is reduced to one half of a cup. Strain this out and let it cool. Add one fourth of a cup of raw, organic apple cider vinegar to the sage and chamomile decoction. Apple cider vinegar works well to tone and nourish the skin. Stir this until the two liquids are blended. Add some to a spray bottle and gently mist your clean face up to twice daily. Store this in the refrigerator between uses.

### ACNE-FIGHTING TEA

Beautiful skin starts on the inside. Oftentimes, bad skin is the result of a bad diet. If you struggle with acne, avoid dairy products because they tend to affect the skin. In addition, avoid processed foods and sugars. Cleansing and purifying your body can help treat and prevent acne by flushing out the toxins that cause issues. Yellow dock root is one of the best herbs for this. It is purifying and detoxifying. Try infusing one teaspoon of chopped and dried yellow dock roots into one cup of hot water for ten to fifteen minutes. Drink this up to twice daily for detoxification and purification. Clean up your diet and try to eat more leafy greens as well. If you can do this, you will start to notice your skin glowing with health and vibrancy.

### ACNE WASH

Pau d' arco is an excellent antimicrobial and antibiotic bark, making it perfect for external use treating acne. Create an infusion with this bark by adding one teaspoon of the dried bark to one cup of hot water. Let this infuse for fifteen to twenty minutes. Add one teaspoon of raw honey when the liquid is still warm (but not hot or it will kill the medicinal components in the honey). Allow this to blend into it well. Raw honey is highly antimicrobial and can further help to kill bacteria on the skin's surface. Soak a clean cloth into this mixture and wring it out. Gently wash your clean face with this wash two to three times a day to keep your skin healthy and bacteria-free. This makes enough for several uses, just be sure to store the remainder in the refrigerator between uses.

## Aging

### Anti-Aging Tea 1

The key to keeping skin young is to nourish it with antioxidants. Antioxidant herbs can help to fight free radicals on the skin, which are known for causing damage and aging. A great antioxidant herb to start with is burdock root. This root is utilized in herbal medicine for its powerful antioxidant effects. Infuse one teaspoon of dried and chopped burdock roots into one cup of hot water and let this sit for ten minutes before consuming. Drink one cup daily to keep your skin looking youthful and radiant.

### Anti-Aging Tea 2

Irish Sea Moss is packed full of vitamins and minerals, making it a favorite among those who wish to keep young and healthy. Infuse one half of a teaspoon of Irish Sea moss powder into one cup of hot water and let his blend together well. Add raw honey to taste if you like. Drink one to two cups of this today to nourish your body and integumentary system with vital nutrients that help promote healthy and vitality. Irish Sea moss can also be made into a paste by adding a small amount of water to a teaspoon of the powder. Blend this until it reaches a paste-like consistency and spread it evenly on the facial skin. Leave it for fifteen to twenty minutes before rinsing off to give your skin a boost.

## Allergies

### Allergy Relief Tea

For a daily tea that helps to cleanse the blood and relieve the buildup of histamines that lead to allergies, try sarsaparilla. Sarsaparilla is excellent for allergies because it also lowers inflammation in the body. Inflammation is a major issue for those who suffer from allergies. Infuse one teaspoon of sarsaparilla into one cup of hot water and let this sit for ten minutes before consuming. Drink this daily to keep the blood purified and inflammation at bay.

### Quick Allergy Tea

Quercetin is a compound found in certain plants and herbs that works fast to target inflammation and allergies. There are many plants that contain this beneficial compound, but one of the best and most common are elderberries. Make a strong tea with dried elderberries by infusing one teaspoon in one cup of hot water for fifteen minutes. Adding local raw honey to this tea can also help fight allergies. Drink up to three cups of this tea daily to help fight allergy symptoms like nasal congestion and inflammation, as well as excess mucous.

## FLOWER DECOCTION

Linden flowers are excellent for calming the mind and body, but they can also lower inflammation, making them ideal for allergies. When suffering from allergies, the mucous membranes often become inflamed and can worsen symptoms. Prevent this with a decoction made from linden flowers. Boil two cups of water on the stove and add one half cup of fresh linden flowers or one fourth cup of dried linden flowers. Let this simmer until the liquid is reduced to one cup. Remove this from heat and allow it to cool a little before consuming. You may choose to add some local raw honey to this tea to help further fight allergy symptoms. Drink one cup of this daily to lower inflammation from allergies.

## NETTLE TEA

Stinging nettle contains flavonoids that help to lower histamine production in the body. This is great news for those with allergies, as histamines are to blame for allergy symptoms and the response the body has to allergens. Infuse one teaspoon of dried stinging nettle leaves in one cup of hot water and let this sit for seven minutes before consuming. Drink one cup daily for maintenance or three cups daily for severe allergies.

## *Anemia*

### ANEMIA TEA

Anemia can occur when the body has low iron levels. Thankfully, there is a very common alkaline herb that naturally contains high levels of iron. This herb is the dandelion. The root of the dandelion is often used for blood cleansing and purification, but it is also a valuable source of iron for those in need of higher iron levels to treat anemia. You can create a tea for anemia by infusing one teaspoon of dried and chopped dandelion roots in one cup of hot water. Let this infuse for at least ten minutes to ensure the iron is getting into the tea sufficiently. Drink one to two cups of this tea daily to help increase iron levels and cleans the blood.

## *Arthritis*

### ARTHRITIS MILDING TEA

Kalawalla makes a great addition to a daily routine for the management of arthritis, especially rheumatoid arthritis. It works to balance the immune system and help keep it from attacking the body. It is great for a variety of autoimmune conditions for this reason. Infuse one teaspoon of dried kalawalla leaves in one cup of hot water for seven minutes before consuming. Drink one cup daily to keep the immune system balanced and prevent immune system attacks on the joints.

### QUICK ANALGESIC ARTHRITIS TEA

Chaparral is highly anti-inflammatory and analgesic, making it ideal for treating pain from arthritis. It you happen to find yourself in need of quick relief, try making a strong tea with chaparral. Infuse one teaspoon of the aerial parts of the plant into one cup of very hot water. Let this sit and infuse for ten to fifteen minutes. Drink this when it has cooled enough to comfortably consume. Drink up to two cups of this daily for arthritis pain relief. Try using the arthritis ointment detailed below in conjunction with this remedy for maximum pain relief.

### ARTHRITIS OINTMENT

Soursop leaves can be used externally to bring relief to arthritic joints. They work to reduce inflammation that results from arthritis. Reducing inflammation means reducing pain in the area. These leaves can be applied like a poultice to the areas, or you can make an ointment to use any time you need it. To do this, start by infusing dried soursop leaves in a carrier oil. Olive oil makes a great carrier oil for this, as it is nourishing to the skin and can soothe any skin issues caused by arthritis. Let this infuse for four to six weeks in a dark place. Shake your soursop and oil blend daily to promote further infusion. After four to six weeks, strain out the oil and put eight ounces of this in a double boiler. Under low heat, add one ounce of beeswax (preferably grated beeswax or beeswax pellets). Let the beeswax melt into the oil infusion completely and then turn off the heat. You may choose at this time to add ten to twenty drops of essential oils like peppermint, eucalyptus, turmeric, ginger, or copaiba. These help manage pain. Pour the ointment into jars to cool. When it cools, it will take on a salve-like consistency that is easy to apply to any area you choose and stays in place. Use this ointment as often as you need for relief from sore muscles, joints, and areas of trauma. As with any salve, avoid getting it in the eyes or mucous membranes.

## Asthma

### QUICK ACTING ASTHMA TEA

If you find it hard to take a deep breath and are in need of quick relief, you can create a tea that can help to calm the body and open the airways fast. Two alkaline herbs that help with this are mullein and eucalyptus. Mullein is great for clearing the airways of mucous, especially the bronchial passages. Eucalyptus also helps to open the airways and promote respiratory health. It contains a constituent called 1,8 cineole that has been shown in studies to decrease anxiety before operations, which means it may help to calm the body when it is experiencing issues with asthma as well. Combine one teaspoon each of mullein and eucalyptus in one cup of very hot water. Let these infuse for at least five minutes. While you are waiting, it helps to lean down and inhale the steam coming off the tea. This can open airways and calm the body, even before you consume it. When it has sufficiently cooled, consume the tea, pausing between sips to focus on breathing. Do this as often as needed to cope with asthma.

### SOOTHING TEA

To soothe the body and calm spasmodic issues with the lungs and airways, try a tea made with mugwort. Mugwort is antispasmodic and anti-inflammatory, making it ideal for treating asthma or related conditions of the respiratory system. Its nervine properties mean it can calm anxiety that leads to asthmatic conditions. If you feel like you are stressed or overwhelmed, these may trigger an asthma attack. When you start to feel this way, make a cup of mugwort tea. Infuse one teaspoon of dried mugwort leaves into one cup of hot water for up to seven minutes. Consume this when it has cooled sufficiently. You can drink up to 2 cups daily, as needed, for soothing relief from asthmatic conditions.

## *Autism*

## Remedies

### AUTISTIC TREATMENT

Detox the body of mucus by proper blood flow that supply oxygen to the brain. It is a neurological condition. The brain works differently, and in the case of epilepsy there is abnormal nerve cell activity in the brain.

## *Back Pain*

### SPINE'S FINE TINCTURE

Mullein is often known for the medicinal properties in its leaves and flowers. However, mullein root holds a powerful medicinal secret: it can soothe spasmodic conditions relating to back and spine pain. It is an excellent remedy for any musculoskeletal issue, ranging from back muscles to a bruised coccyx. The root is best prepared in a tincture for spine pain. Start by harvesting mullein roots and chopping them. Fill a glass jar with the chopped roots and then completely cover them in at least 80 proof alcohol. Let this sit and infuse for four to six weeks. Keep this out of direct sunlight and in a cool, dark place while it infuses. Shake this daily (make sure the lid is on good) to help the mullein root further infuse into the alcohol solvent. After four to six weeks, strain out the tincture and bottle it. It is best to store tinctures in dropper bottles if possible. Take two to three droppers full as needed when you are feeling back pain coming on.

### WARMING COMPRESS

Sometimes one of the best ways to combat back pain is by using a warming compress. The heat, blended with the medicinal properties in the herbal compress, helps to gently soothe and ease away pain. Guaco leaves make an excellent remedy in a compress for back pain. Start your compress by boiling one ounce of dried guaco leaves in three to four cups of water on the stove. Turn down the heat then let this simmer for fifteen to twenty minutes. Take the pot off of heat and set it aside to cool. Let this cool enough to where it doesn't hurt when the liquid is applied to the skin. When the liquid is still warm, soak a clean rag in it until it is fully soaked. Wring it out a little then place it on your back where you are experiencing pain. Let this sit on the area for as long as you can. Try lying down on your stomach when you are treating yourself with this remedy. Repeat as often as needed.

### SCIATIC PAIN TEA

Sciatic pain comes from a nerve called the sciatic nerve. Sciatic nerve goes from your lower back through the hips to the leg. When it is aggravated, it can cause a shooting pain that radiates through these areas. To effectively tackle pain in this nerve, you will need herbs that act on the nerves. These are called "nervines." Some effective nervine herbs include blue vervain and mugwort. They act on the nervous system to calm the nerves and reduce pain. They can help with pain, inflammation, and tension as well. To make this nervine tea, combine one teaspoon each of blue vervain and mugwort and infuse them in one cup of hot water for up to seven minutes. Consume this when it is cool enough to comfortably drink. Drink one to two cups daily for help with nerve pain and spasms.

### ANALGESIC DAILY TEA FOR BACK PAIN

A tea made with chamomile and elder is ideal for pain relief when it comes to back pain, spasms, and inflammation. Elderberry is very anti-inflammatory and can help reduce any inflammation that may be leading to pain. Chamomile is antispasmodic and calming. It can help reduce any tension that is causing pain. Together, these two alkaline herbs are perfect for back pain caused by inflammation and/or tension. They are gentle enough to use in a daily tea for overall health. To create this healing tea, combine one teaspoon each of chamomile flowers and dried elderberries. Let them infuse in one cup of hot water for seven to ten minutes before consuming. Drink one cup daily to support and nourish your back.

### SOOTHING BACK PAIN TEA

Hops and blue vervain are known for their effect on the body and mind. Hops (also called lupulo) are sedative and anti-inflammatory. They can calm tension, as well as reduce inflammation that causes back pain. Blue vervain works on the nerves to calm spasms, reduce pain, and calm tension. Together, these provide soothing support for those experiencing any kind of back pain. Add one teaspoon of each herb to a tea bag and let this infuse in one cup of hot water for five to seven minutes before consuming. Do this daily for back pain and inflammation maintenance, or as needed when you are experiencing extra tension and stress due to back pain.

## Bedsores

### BEDSORE TOPICAL WASH

Bedsores result when skin becomes damaged due to decreased blood flow to the area over a period of time. This usually happens when someone is immobile and cannot move to circulate blood to all areas of the body as it should. Damaged skin from poor circulation to the area will appear as an ulcer on the skin or an infected, inflamed area. They are often sore and very painful. Alkaline herbs to treat these include chickweed and yarrow. Chickweed will provide soothing relief to the area, helping to reduce redness and inflammation. Yarrow helps to cleanse the wound and promote healing. These two works synergistically to tackle bedsores in different ways. Create an effective topical wash with chickweed and yarrow to treat bedsores by first boiling two to three cups of water on the stove. Add one ounce each of chickweed (preferably fresh) and yarrow (leaves and flowers if possible). Reduce heat and let this simmer for twenty minutes, or until the liquid is reduced by half. Wait until this has completely cooled before using it. You can use it in two ways: as a topical wash or compress. For a topical wash, simply wash the bedsores with this liquid up to five times daily. For a compress, soak a clean rag in the liquid and place it on the affected areas twice daily. In between compresses, wash and cleanse the wounds with the liquid as well. If at all possible, try to get movement and circulation to the area by moving the body as much as possible. A poultice of raw honey also works on bedsores to cleanse and heal the wounds, and is especially effective when used in conjunction with the topical wash.

## *Bronchitis*

### FIRE CIDER

Fire cider is an age-old remedy that employs heat from a variety of natural herbs to target viruses and infections. There are many different recipes for fire cider in different regions of the world, but many contain the following ingredients: turmeric, ginger, onion, garlic, cayenne peppers, jalapeno peppers, horseradish root, rosemary, thyme, sage, and lemon.

This colorful creation is infused in raw, organic apple cider vinegar for maximum potency. Chop one turmeric and one ginger root, one onion, one garlic bulb, one horseradish root, three to five cayenne or jalapeno peppers, one lemon, and two to three large cuttings of fresh rosemary, thyme, and sage. Fill a glass jar with these ingredients and completely cover them in apple cider vinegar to infuse.

Let this sit in a cool, dark place for at least one month before straining it out. Take a shot glass full (one ounce) as needed when you feel like you are coming down with a virus. It will heat up the body and kill infection or pathogens that are causing sickness.

### THROAT SOOTHING TEA

Sage is an herb often used for its soothing and antimicrobial properties. It comes in especially handy for throat issues. If you are experiencing any drainage that irritates the throat, try a tea made with sage. Infuse one teaspoon of sage leaves (fresh or dried) into one cup of hot water. Let this infuse for five minutes. Adding one teaspoon of raw honey to this tea maximizes the throat soothing action of the tea and further helps to heal a sore throat. Drink this up to three times daily when you have a sore throat.

### SWEET SOOTHING TEA

For a soothing tea that helps to open the airways and prevents infection, try a tea made with mullein leaves and pau d' arco bark. Together, these alkaline herbs help to prevent infections like pneumonia, while soothing irritation and inflammation in the respiratory system. They will also help the body expel any excess mucous causing issues. Infuse one teaspoon each of mullein leaves and pau d' arco bark into one cup of hot water. Let this sit for seven minutes before consuming. Add raw honey to sweeten this tea, as well as provide antimicrobial action. Drink one to three cups daily to help treat bronchitis while preventing any infections that may result from the excess mucous in the airways.

## *Burns and Sunburns*

### BURN HEALING HONEY

Honey works wonders for all kinds of wounds, so it is no surprise it makes an excellent sunburn treatment. Maximize the treatment by infusing soothing chickweed into the honey. After harvesting chickweed, let it wilt for twenty-four hours and then place it in a glass jar. Cover the chickweed in raw, unfiltered honey. Let this infuse indefinitely. Use it as needed by applying a small amount to the affected areas and reapplying as needed for cooling comfort and healing.

## SUNBURN SPRAY

A sunburn spray is a very effective way to reach sunburn on your back because you can get the spray to reach the area. Create a soothing spray by boiling one cup of water with one teaspoon of chickweed until the liquid is reduced by half. Blend this with one half cup of aloe vera juice. Aloe vera is one of the best cures for sunburn because it is cooling, anti-inflammatory, and restorative to the skin. Store this in the refrigerator between uses. Spray on sunburned areas for instant relief.

## BURN POULTICE

For burns that begin to blister, a poultice may be the best route for treatment. Create a quick poultice by grinding up fresh chickweed and add a little aloe vera juice to give it a paste-like consistency. Together, chickweed and aloe vera will provide a soothing, cooling sensation while working to heal redness, inflammation, and irritation. Apply this evenly to the affected areas and leave it on as long as possible. Repeat if possible, up to three times daily.

## IMMUNITY STRENGTHENER

For a strong immune system, try making a glycerite or tincture with elderberries. The berries are immunomodulators, meaning they can help keep the immune system running strong and healthy. They have been shown in studies to boost the immune system when it is exposed to a virus, as well as help the body fight off viruses more effectively. To make a tincture, fill a jar with dried berries and then completely cover them in at least 80 proof alcohol. If you happen to have any cinnamon sticks, add a few to this for extra immune strengthening power. Let this site and infuse in a cool, dark place for four to six weeks. After four to six weeks, strain everything out and bottle it. Take five milliliters up to four times daily at the first sign of sickness or if you have been exposed to someone you later find out was sick. To make a glycerite, fill a jar with dried or fresh elderberries and a little cinnamon if you have it. Completely cover the elderberries in non-GMO food grade vegetable glycerin. Let this infuse for four to six weeks, shaking daily to help infuse. After four to six weeks, pour the entire contents of the jar in a pot on the stove under low heat. Let this come to a boil slowly. After it has come to a boil, reduce the heat and let this sit on low heat for up to six hours. Keep an eye on your pot and stir as needed. Let this cool and strain it out through a cheesecloth, making sure to squeeze the cheesecloth hard to get the trapped liquid out. Bottle this and take five to ten milliliters at the first sign of sickness or if you believe you have been exposed to sickness.

## Canker Sores

### ANTI-INFLAMMATORY MOUTHWASH

For stubborn and bothersome canker sores, try a mouthwash with pau d' arco and soursop leaves. Pau d' arco will attack any infection or bacteria in the mouth, while soursop leaves help to reduce irritation and inflammation. Make a strong tea with one teaspoon each of dried soursop leaves and pau d' arco bark. Infuse these in a cup of hot water (almost boiling) for ten to twenty minutes. Add one half teaspoon of sea salt or Himalayan salt. Blend this together until the salt has dissolved into the liquid.

When this has sufficiently cooled, gargle fifteen milliliters for up to two minutes. Repeat this up to five times daily to get rid of a canker sore. Store your mouthwash in the refrigerator between uses.

## Cold Sores

### COLD SORE COMPRESS

Cold sores are the result of a virus, so antiviral herbs are required to treat them. An effective herb for the job is linden flower. Linden flowers have been effectively used to treat viruses over the span of time. They are also great for soothing the affected area and reducing redness. Create a strong decoction by boiling one ounce of linden flowers in two cups of water on the stove. Reduce the heat to simmer and let the liquid reduce to one cup. When this has sufficiently cooled, soak a clean rag in the liquid and apply it to the cold sore. Leave this on for up to one hour and reapply as needed until the cold sore is gone. If possible, sleep with a compress by lying on your back to sleep.

### COLD SORE BALM

A combination of yarrow, lemon balm, and St. John's wort work together to eliminate cold sores quickly. Infuse one part of each herb in coconut oil. Warm the coconut oil first by sitting the jar in a pan of warm water. When enough has melted to cover the plant material, pour it in the jar. Next, place the glass jar of herbs and coconut oil in a pan of hot water on the stove. If you have a "warm" setting on your stove, this works perfectly. If not, try sitting it in a pan of hot water on a burner under very low heat. Let this infuse for up to twelve hours before straining it out. In a double boiler, add eight ounces of herb-infused coconut oil to one ounce of beeswax. Let the beeswax melt thoroughly and then pour the balm into jars to cool. This can easily be applied to cold sores to treat them effectively and rapidly. Each herb used attacks viruses at their source and helps to quickly heal the irritated skin. Use this balm at the very first sign of a cold sore for best results. Use it as often as you can when you feel one coming.

### COLD SORE TEA

A tea made with elderflower and Echinacea can work to boost the immune system to help the body fight off the herpes virus responsible for cold sores. Elder flowers work much like elderberries to fight viruses and infections. Echinacea helps to boost the immune system and stop a virus in its tracks. Infuse one teaspoon each of elderflower and Echinacea in one cup of hot water for five to seven minutes. Consume one to three cups daily to treat a cold sore. Use this tea in conjunction with the cold sore balm for an even faster recovery.

### COLD SORE MOUTHWASH

An antiviral and soothing mouthwash made from pau d' arco and soursop leaves can help to treat, as well as prevent, cold sores. Pau d' arco is antiviral in addition to antimicrobial. Soursop leaves are highly anti-inflammatory. They can work to reduce any swelling or mouth irritation caused by cold sores. Infuse one teaspoon each of soursop leaves and pau d' arco in one cup of boiling water. Let this simmer for fifteen minutes until the liquid is reduced by half. Remove this from heat and add a pinch of sea salt or Himalayan salt. Let this dissolve into the liquid. Allow the mouthwash to cool completely before using it. Gargle fifteen milliliters for up to two minutes in your mouth to help treat cold sores. Repeat this up to three times daily. Use the cold sore balm in conjunction with this remedy for rapid healing.

## Constipation

### Bowel-Hydrating Infusion

Cascara Sagrada stands in a category by itself when it comes to constipation relief. It hydrates the bowels like no other plant can by promoting excess water in the body to be absorbed by any stool in the bowels. An increase of water in the stool causes it to increase in volume and push its way out of the body easier. You can create a gentle infusion with this plant to help with constipation by first boiling two cups of water on the stove. Set aside a glass jar filled with two tablespoons of cascara sagrada. Carefully pour the boiling water over the cascara sagrada in the jar and let this sit for one to three hours. Strain out the infusion and Drink one cup when you are in need of relief. Wait at least one hour. If you do not see any results, drink the other cup (the recipe makes two cups). Make sure to drink a lot of water when you are taking this infusion, as it pulls water from the body and may result in dehydration if you do not keep drinking water to hydrate yourself.

### Bowel-Motivating Tincture

Sometimes the bowels can be stubborn and need something to get them moving correctly. Healthy bowels start with a healthy diet, so make sure you are eating a clean diet full of alkaline foods. Avoid processed foods and sugars. You can also help things along with a tincture made from mugwort and cascara sagrada. Fill a jar with one part cascara sagrada and two parts mugwort. Cover the plant material completely with at least 80 proof alcohol. Let this sit in a cool, dark place for four to six weeks, making sure to shake daily to help it infuse better. After four to six weeks, strain out the tincture and bottle it. Take one to three droppers full when you are feeling constipated. Wait six hours before taking more. Repeat as needed for relief from constipation.

### Bowel-Soothing Tea

For a tea that helps to soothe irritated bowels and an upset stomach, try infusing chamomile and sage in a cup of hot water. Use one teaspoon each of chamomile and sage and let them infuse for up to ten minutes. Chamomile is famous for its calming and soothing effects on the stomach and bowels sage is carminative as well. Try adding a little raw honey to sweeten the tea and lend its gentle healing properties to the blend. Drink one to three cups daily for help with bowel and stomach discomfort.

### Purifying Digestive Tea

For bowels in need of cleansing and purification, use dandelion and burdock root. Dandelion root is a great tonic for the body and can help flush out toxins. In addition to the root, the leaves are a powerful bitter herb. Add one half teaspoon of dried roots and one half teaspoon of dried leaves to this tea blend. Add one teaspoon of burdock root as well. Burdock root is cleansing and purifying. It helps flush out impurities and promote healthy digestion. Infuse these herbs in one cup of hot water for up to ten minutes. Drink one to two cups of this tea as needed for digestive purification.

## Cough and Cold

### LUNG LUBRICATING TEA

Sometimes a cough can leave your lungs feeling irritated, inflamed, and sore. For a tea that helps to lubricate and nourish the respiratory tract, try marshmallow root and mugwort tea. Marshmallow root is known for its ability to lubricate irritated membranes in the body. It is soothing and cooling. Mugwort's nervine and anti-inflammatory properties help to further provide relief for tired lungs. Combine one teaspoon of marshmallow root and one teaspoon of mugwort in one cup of hot water. Let this sit for ten minutes before consuming. Drink one to three cups daily to help heal and repair the lungs.

### ANTITUSSIVE OXYMEL

A combination of sage and wild bergamot help to quiet a bothersome cough. When infused in honey and apple cider vinegar to make an oxymel, you have a powerful healing cough treatment. An oxymel is generally an herbal preparation made with raw honey and apple cider vinegar. It is antimicrobial, healing, and antitussive. Sage is anti-spasomdic, making it perfect for calming a spasmodic cough. Wild bergamot is native to much of North America and grows wild and in abundance in many areas. The flower heads and leaves are full of powerful therapeutic properties, including antimicrobial, anti-inflammatory, and antibiotic attributes. They have a similar chemical composition to thyme, which is also a powerful cold and cough remedy. To create an oxymel with these herbs, fill a glass jar with one part wild bergamot leaves and flowers and one part sage leaves. Fill the jar, covering the plant material halfway. Cover the plant material the rest of the way with apple cider vinegar. Shake this well and store it in a cool, dry place to infuse. Shake the jar daily to help the plants infuse into the honey and apple cider vinegar better. Let this infuse for up to one month before straining it out. Take ten to fifteen milliliters as needed to calm a stubborn cough.

### COUGH SYRUP

If you are in need of a quick and effective cough syrup, this recipe is perfect. This cough syrup recipe is especially helpful for those times you wake up in the night with a cough (or someone in your household is keeping you awake with a cough) and you need to whip something together to help fast. Start by filling a small cup with one teaspoon of raw honey. Add a half teaspoon of ground ginger and a fourth teaspoon of ground cinnamon. Next, add a squeeze of lemon juice and one half teaspoon of raw organic apple cider vinegar. Blend these ingredients together well. Take ten milliliters as needed to help control a cough, soothe the throat, and fight a cold.

### SOOTHING COUGH AND COLD FORMULA

For help with a spasmodic cough that has you feeling drained and weary, try a formula with yarrow and hops. This blend is also great for fighting a cold or virus. Yarrow is often used for viruses because it induces sweating and helps to purge the body of toxins while lowering any fever. Hops is known for its soothing and nervine properties, making it effective for calming the body and helping bring much needed rest to aid in recovery. Add one part yarrow and one part hops to a glass jar and cover half of the plant material with at least 80 proof alcohol. Cover the plant material the rest of the way with raw honey and shake this well. Store this in a cool, dry place for one month and strain it out through a strainer. Take five to ten milliliters of this formula up to four times daily as needed for help with a cough or virus that has you feeling down.

## Lakota Cough and Cold Formula

The Lakota Indians used wild bergamot, or Monarda fistulosa, as a powerful cough and cold remedy. Studies show this plant to be highly antimicrobial and antiviral. It contains high amounts of the compound thymol, making it a strong therapeutic remedy for coughs and colds. To get the most out of this plant, try making a formula that extracts both the alcohol and water soluble properties from the plant. First, fill a jar with fresh or dried wild bergamot flowers and leaves. Cover the plant material with 80 proof alcohol and let this infuse for four to six weeks in a cool, dark place. Save some wild bergamot leaves and flowers to make a strong decoction on the stove. Boil two cups of water and add one ounce of wild bergamot. Let this simmer until the liquid is reduced by half. Strain it out and let it cool. Strain out the tincture and combine even amounts of the tincture and decoction in a jar. Add a small amount of raw honey for taste. Take ten milliliters of this formula at the first sign of sickness or coughing.

## Lumbee Cough and Cold Formula

A sacred plant that grew in the North Carolina region was highly esteemed by the Lumbee Indians. This plant is goldenseal. Today, this plant is still highly revered by herbalists and natural healers. It is a source of the healing compound berberine, which is thought to combat upper respiratory infections and many other types of infections in the body. Goldenseal is endangered or threatened in some areas of the country and should be sustainably harvested to ensure its survival. If possible, it is best cultivated for use instead of wildcrafted. To make a strong formula with goldenseal, you will need the roots and aerial parts of the plant. These both contain compounds that complement one another and help the body absorb the medicinal compounds in the plant easier. Fill a glass jar with one part roots and one part leaves from the goldenseal plant.

Completely cover the plant material with at least 80 proof alcohol and let this infuse for four to six weeks in a cool, dark place. Strain out the liquid and store this in a dropper bottle. For a cough or respiratory infection, take one to three droppers full in a glass of warm water with one teaspoon of raw honey. Repeat this as needed to treat and prevent respiratory infections.

## Quick Acting Cough and Cold Formula

For a formula that tackles cough and congestion fast, try a combination of mullein, yarrow, and elderberry. Mullein is one of the best and most effective herbs for treating respiratory issues. It can help clear the airways and expel excess mucous. Yarrow is antimicrobial and febrifuge, making it useful for colds and viruses.

Elderberry can strengthen the immune system and help the body fight off any infection or virus. Together, these three herbs work synergistically to promote a fast recovery. Add one part mullein leaves, one part yarrow leaves, and one part elderberry to a glass jar. Cover half the plant material with at least 80 proof alcohol and cover the rest of the plant material with raw honey. Shake the formula well to blend the honey and alcohol. Let this infuse in a cool, dark place for four to six weeks, shaking it daily to promote infusion. When the four to six weeks are up, strain out the liquid and bottle it. Take five to ten milliliters as needed to combat a cough or virus.

## EXPECTORATING COUGH AND COLD TEA

To get rid of the excess mucous that comes with a cough or cold, try a combination of mullein and guaco. Mullein will bring the mucous out of the airways and guaco will reduce inflammation that holds mucous in the airways, as well as relieve spasms that cause coughing. Infuse one teaspoon of mullein leaves and one teaspoon of guaco leaves in one cup of hot water for seven minutes. Add raw honey to taste (it is also good for coughs). Drink one to three dups daily to promote the removal of excess mucous from the lungs and bronchial passages.

## DECONGESTANT TEA

For a tea to combat congestion, an effective combination of eucalyptus and pleurisy root can help. Eucalyptus opens the airways and promotes healthy bronchial passages. Pleurisy root has been used for centuries by indigenous people to help drain excess fluid from the lungs, preventing pneumonia and any lung infection. It is invaluable to help keep the lungs healthy and able to breathe clearly. Pleurisy root is a root from a common North American plant often called by the common name "butterfly weed." Combine one teaspoon of dried and chopped pleurisy root and one teaspoon of eucalyptus leaves. Infuse these in one cup of hot water for five to seven minutes. Drink this tea up to three times daily to keep the lungs and bronchial passages clear of fluid and mucous.

## ANTITUSSIVE FLOWER TEA

For a gentle floral tea blend to combat spasmodic coughing, try elderflower and chamomile. Elderflower is antiviral and anti-inflammatory. Chamomile flowers are anti-spasmodic and nervine. They can help prevent coughing and calm the body. Infuse one teaspoon of each flower in one cup of hot water for seven minutes. Add some raw honey to make a delicious, sweet floral flavor. Drink one to three cups of this tea daily if you are in need of help to calm a cough.

## Cramps

## MUSCLE WARMING OINTMENT

For an ointment that gently warms, try drying powder of St. John's wort. St. John's wort is one of the most popular medicinal herbs for helping with muscular pain, headaches, arthritis, asthma, cough, cramps, flu, cold, sexual issues, high blood pressure, migraines, morning sickness, menopausal symptoms, PMS, sciatica, and much more. Compared to other remedies, it is also easily available, and very economical. All you need to do is buy the ointment or gel that combines st. John's and the dried powder. You can put it on your skin or mix it into a bar so it can be carried around. You can also snack on it when you need it. Just mix the powder in hot water and drink it three times daily.

## MUSCLE CRAMP TEA

Eucalyptus is a plant known for its pleasant aroma and range of therapeutic properties. If you have a mild muscle cramp, make a tea from eucalyptus for an affordable and simple aid to relax those muscles. Eucalyptus has been used as a pain reliever as well as a diaphoretic since ancient times. In fact, eucalyptus oil, distilled from the leaves, is used as a staple ingredient for many cough and cold remedies. To make an excellent eucalyptus tea for treating muscle cramp, add three to five grams to your cup and add it to hot water. You can sweeten with honey to make it tasty and make it more effective in treating muscle cramps and pain. Drink the tea three times daily to help relieve muscle cramps and prevent them. Rosemary also helps with muscle cramps and can be used in much the same way.

## MUSCLE RUB

For external pain relief, eucalyptus can be made into a powerful muscle rub that treats sore muscles and joints. Start by filling a sterile glass jar with dried eucalyptus leaves. Completely cover the leaves in a carrier oil like olive oil. Sit this somewhere to infuse for four to six weeks. Shake it daily. Keep the jar out of direct sunlight to prevent damaging the plant material and making it less potent. After four to six weeks, strain out the oil and add eight ounces to a double boiler. Next, add one ounce of beeswax and let this melt under low heat. Remove the muscle rub mixture from heat when the beeswax melts. At this time, you may choose to increase the potency even more by adding ten to twenty drops of eucalyptus, peppermint, tea tree, or rosemary essential oil, but this is optional. Pour the muscle rub into jars to cool. Apply a liberal amount of this to sore muscles and joints as needed.

## *Diarrhea*

## ASTRINGENT TEA

Yarrow is an alkaline herb that has astringent properties, making it useful to bring relief to the bowels by encouraging the healing of the intestines and tissues that are irritated. Astringent herbs tighten tissues and tone weak body tissue. When one has diarrhea, the intestines may be weak and in need of toning astringents. Additionally, astringent herbs help reduce irritation, redness, and swelling. They are often used to treat complaints like diarrhea, hemorrhoids, and inflammatory conditions. Make a gentle and soothing tea with yarrow leaves or flowers by infusing one teaspoon of yarrow in one cup of hot water for five to seven minutes. Drink two to three cups as needed for astringent healing. This tea can also be used as a wash to treat hemorrhoids. If using it as a hemorrhoid wash, cleanse the affected area up to five times daily with this tea recipe.

## CINNAMON POWDER CAPSULES

Cinnamon is a rich source of a compound called coumarin. This medicinal compound has many uses, including lowering inflammation, nourishing the heart, easing digestive woes, killing bacteria and viruses, increasing circulation, and eliminating fungal infections. For digestive complaints like diarrhea, cinnamon can help stimulate salivation and gastric juices which in turn can ease digestion. Many people opt to take cinnamon daily as a dietary supplement for many ailments, so they grind it into powder to put in capsules. It is important to note that not all cinnamon is created equal. There are two varieties: cassia cinnamon and Ceylon cinnamon. Cassia is what most people use and is more readily available at grocery stores. Ceylon is considered "true" cinnamon. It has a sweeter flavor and less coumarin. You might think that less coumarin is bad since coumarin is also what gives cinnamon its medicinal properties. However, too much coumarin is not safe because it can result in liver damage if taken over time. In higher doses, coumarin can also thin the blood too much. Ceylon has just the right amount of coumarin to be safe and effective. Place 150 milligrams of Ceylon cinnamon powder into capsules and take two daily for help with diarrhea and stomach complaints.

## QUICK AND EASY DIARRHEA TEA

An alkaline herb that has been shown to be very effective for treating diarrhea is stinging nettle. Stinging nettle not only helps replenish vital nutrients the body may be lacking from diarrhea, but it can help eliminate diarrhea and return your intestinal tract to normal. For many people with chronic diarrhea, they may find they are lacking in nutrients that keep them healthy and balanced. Stinging nettle is a rich and robust source of vitamins A, C, K, and B. They also contain valuable minerals and fatty acids. A tea made with stinging nettle is the perfect remedy to balance the body, replenish lost nutrients, and encourage a healthy intestinal tract after suffering from diarrhea. Make a strong tea so you get all the nutrients by infusing two teaspoons of stinging nettle into one cup of hot water for ten minutes. Drink these two to three times daily for the treatment and prevention of diarrhea. Make sure to drink plenty of water if you have diarrhea, as it can dehydrate the body fast.

## SOOTHING DIARRHEA TEA

Chamomile and Sage are soothing to the stomach and intestinal tract, so they are the perfect alkaline remedy for treating diarrhea, an upset stomach, gas, bloating, and a wide variety of stomach and intestinal ailments. Chamomile's soothing and anti-spasmodic properties make it perfect for calming a spasmodic gut when you have diarrhea. Sage works to calm the digestive tract as well, and can help bring quick relief when you need it. Combine one teaspoon each of chamomile flowers and sage leaves in one cup of hot water. Let this infuse for five to seven minutes before enjoying. Drink one to three cups as needed for the treatment of diarrhea, upset stomach, gas, bloating, or other similar digestive complaints.

## IROQUOIS TEA

Agrimony is a native plant to much of North America. This beneficial plant was used by the Iroquois to treat stomach complaints and especially diarrhea. All parts of the agrimony plant were used to heal the body. This plant is easy to find in the summer months and is identified by its yellow flowers that emerge on spikes. When harvesting agrimony, try to take mostly aerial parts to give plants a chance to live. In areas where there are many, you can dig up a few roots to use medicinally as well. Process the plants by cleaning them and then laying or hanging them to dry. Store the dried plants in an airtight jar and keep them out of direct sunlight. This way you will have plenty of good quality agrimony to use when you need it. To make a tea with agrimony, grind up one teaspoon of root and aerial parts of the plant. Infuse this in a cup of hot water for seven to ten minutes before consuming it. Drink one to three cups of this tea daily or as needed for the treatment of diarrhea and other digestive complaints.

*Fatigue*

### SHAKE-IT-OFF FORMULA

If you are being held back by mild to moderate depression, try a formula made with damiana and blue vervain to start your day. Those suffering from mild to moderate depression often report that they feel fatigued and tired a lot. They may also experience little to no motivation. Damiana can help to balance hormones that cause fatigue and depression. Blue vervain acts as a nervine to promote feelings of positivity and uplifting. Combine one part damiana and one part blue vervain in a sterile glass jar and completely cover the plant material with at least 80 proof alcohol. Let this infuse for four to six weeks in a cool, dark place. After four to six weeks, strain out the liquid and bottle it in a dropper bottle. Take two to three droppers full in the morning with food. Take one to three droppers full in the afternoon as needed to control depression, fatigue, and low motivation.

### UP AND ABOUT MORSELS

Do you find it hard to get going in the morning? Many people have a hard time getting out of bed and getting their day started. You can help super-charge your body and get off to a great start with Up and About Morsels. These contain Nopal and Irish Sea Moss. Both of these are superfoods. Superfoods are foods that are packed with important vitamins, minerals, and other nutrients to give you optimal nutrition. This nutrition can help you start your day with energy and stamina in order to tackle anything that comes your way. To make these, infuse one tablespoon each of powdered nopal and powdered Irish Sea moss into one cup of organic coconut oil under low heat for one hour. Remove from heat and add one tablespoon of organic, gluten free rolled oats and one tablespoon of organic almond butter. Stir this together well. Place the bowl in the refrigerator for fifteen minutes or until you notice the coconut oil start to go back to a solid state. Before the coconut oil becomes too hard to work with, take it out of the refrigerator and stir the contents of the bowl one more time. Now take a spoonful of the mixture at a time and roll it into a small ball. Place the balls on a flat surface and sit it in the refrigerator overnight to harden completely. Enjoy a cup of these each morning to give you a protein and nutrition boost to enliven your day.

### PICK-ME-UP TEA

If you find yourself needing a pick-me-up as you go about your day, try a purifying and cleansing tea made with burdock root. Burdock root can help flush out the toxins that weigh you down and make you sluggish throughout the day. Infuse one teaspoon of burdock root in one cup of hot water for five to seven minutes. Add a little raw honey to taste (and for an additional pick-me-up). Enjoy one cup of this tea in the afternoon when you feel yourself start to get tired and fatigued after a long day.

## INVIGORATING TEA

Eucalyptus is a lively and invigorating alkaline herb. Its fresh and camphorous compounds help bring energy and vigor to a tired body and mind. It is often enjoyed in the aromatherapy world for its ability to bring energy and vitality just from the scent alone. Drinking it in tea can help give you the momentum you need to get your day going or the vigor to finish the day strong. In addition, it can help open up the sinuses and allow you to breathe easier and deeper. Infuse one teaspoon of eucalyptus leaves into one cup of hot water for five to seven minutes. Add a small amount of raw honey for an extra boost. Drink this in the morning or afternoon for a stimulating and revitalizing experience.

## *Fever*

## FEVER-REDUCING TEA

Yarrow is one of the most popular herbs for reducing a fever. It is known to work by inducing sweating, which helps to naturally cool the body down. You can create a gentle and effective tea for treating high fevers by infusing one teaspoon of dried or fresh yarrow leaves into one cup of hot water for five to seven minutes. Drink one to four cups daily as needed for help reducing a fever. A fever should be left alone unless it gets very high. It is the body's way of heating up to make itself inhospitable for a virus or infection. If you bring a fever down when it is not that high you are robbing yourself of this tactic that is helping to kill a virus or pathogen and heal you. Keep an eye on a fever and take your temperature often when you feel you have a fever. Let the fever get up to 103- or 104- Fahrenheit before you take action. An exception to this rule is if the fever is making you miserable and you are unable to keep food or water down because of it. Drink plenty of fluids when you have a fever to avoid dehydration, as a fever can make one dehydrated faster than normal.

## FEVER-BREAKING TEA

Sarsaparilla is another alkaline herb that works to reduce a fever. It is also a great source of iron, helping to keep you strong and healthy. Create a tea with sarsaparilla by infusing one teaspoon of dried sarsaparilla into one cup of hot water for seven to ten minutes. Drink one to two cups as needed for help controlling a high fever. In addition, consider taking a tepid bath to bring a fever down. Another helpful action you can take to help with a fever is to place a cool compress on the forehead or neck area.

## QUICK-ACTING FEVER TEA

A powerful and synergistic combination of elderberry and yarrow can help manage a fever quickly. These two herbs work to fight illness in two ways: the elderberry stimulates the immune system and helps if fight the cause of the illness while the yarrow helps lower a fever and flush out any toxins that may be causing issues. Infuse one teaspoon of yarrow and one teaspoon of dried elderberries in one cup of hot water for ten minutes. Add raw honey to taste. Drink one to four cups of this tea daily to knock out a fever fast.

*Food Intolerances*

## GUT-HEAL TEA

Sometimes the gut becomes imbalanced and the bad bacteria take over. Keeping our microbiome healthy is of the utmost importance because much of our immune systems rely on a healthy gut biome to function properly. Slippery Elm and Cinnamon can help replenish the good bacteria while promoting regular bowel movements to keep you healthy. Infuse one teaspoon of slippery elm bark and one teaspoon of finely chopped cinnamon bark into one cup of hot water for ten minutes. Stir this well and drink one to two cups of this tea daily to manage gut health, a healthy microbiome, and digestive wellness.

## BUILD-UP BROTH

Stinging Nettle is one of the best alkaline herbs for replenishing the body and providing essential nutrients. If you need built up after an illness, surgery, or diarrhea, try a nourishing broth made with stinging nettle leaves. A combination of the broth and the nutrient-dense nettle leaves will help restore the body and nurture the gut. Making your own bone broth is so much easier than most people realize. The next time you cook a turkey, chicken, beef, or any other meat with bones, try making a broth with the leftover bones. You can do this by filling a large stock pot with the bones and water. Add hearty and nutritious ingredients to the pot like garlic cloves, onions, rosemary, thyme, or sage. Add 1 to 2 cups of fresh or dried stinging nettle leaves to the pot as well. Bring the pot of water, bones, and herbs to a boil and reduce the heat to simmer. Let this simmer for as long as possible to make sure you get all the nourishing collagen from the bones and connective tissues. You can leave the pot simmering under very low heat for up to twelve hours if you want. Just make sure to keep an eye on it so it doesn't evaporate down too much. Pour the finished broth through a strainer and into jars to store. If you won't be using it right away, you can portion it out into containers and freeze some. When you need built-up, simply take some broth out of the freezer and gently re-heat it on the stove. Enjoy this as needed when you are recovering.

## STOP FLATULENCE TEA

Stop uncomfortable gas and bloating with a tea made from chamomile. This alkaline herb both soothes and calms digestive discomfort that leads to gas. Chamomile also calms spasms that cause discomfort in the digestive tract. Make a calming tea by infusing one teaspoon of dried or fresh chamomile flowers into one cup of hot water for five to seven minutes. Drink one to three cups as needed to help with flatulence and digestive woes.

## COLON-SOOTHING TEA

Mugwort has been used for digestive issues for centuries because it is so versatile when it comes to what this herb does for the digestive tract. It is a bitter digestive, meaning it can help manage colic, gas, cramps, constipation, diarrhea, and sluggish digestion. Mugwort makes the perfect herb for colon soothing because of all it can do. Make a comforting tea with mugwort by infusing one teaspoon of dried or fresh mugwort into one cup of hot water for five to seven minutes. Drink this daily for colon health and comfort.

## Hangover

### TAKE-IT-EASY NEXT DAY INFUSION

Replenish lost nutrients from over-indulgence with a strong and nourishing infusion made with stinging nettle. A hangover can leave you dehydrated and in need of sustenance. Stinging nettles can help replace any depleted nutrients while encouraging the flushing of toxins from too much alcohol. This infusion is especially handy if you have a hangover that is causing vomiting or diarrhea. Make an infusion by boiling two cups of water on the stove. Fill a sterile glass jar with one cup of dried or fresh stinging nettle leaves. Carefully pour the boiling water into the glass jar over the stinging nettle. Allow this to sit and infuse for two hours before consuming it. Try to drink the entire infusion by drinking one cup at a time at intervals throughout the day. Drink plenty of water as well.

### NO-FUSS HANGOVER TEA

Dandelion root is an effective remedy for treating a hangover because it helps flush out toxins, cleanses impurities from the body, and acts as a general tonic when you are feeling unwell. In addition, dandelion root can calm an upset stomach, something many people suffering from a hangover experience. Dandelion is very common and easy to come by, so it is an easy remedy when you are feeling down from a hangover. Infuse one teaspoon of chopped (fresh or dried) dandelion root into one cup of water for ten minutes. Add raw honey to taste. Drink 1 to 3 cups of this tea as needed to flush out your system and recover faster. Drink as much water as you can while recovering from a hangover to prevent dehydration and promote cleansing in the body.

### QUICK-ACTING HANGOVER TEA

Sometimes the best cure for a hangover is to stay hydrated and get some rest. Valerian root can help you achieve a deep slumber so you can wake up feeling refreshed and ready to go. Valerian root acts quickly in the body to slow down the Central Nervous System so you can relax and get the rest your body needs. It is also analgesic, so it can calm a headache caused by a hangover. Before consuming, make sure you have consumed plenty of water. When you are ready to lie down and sleep off a hangover, infuse one to two teaspoons of (dried or fresh) chopped valerian root into one cup of hot water. Add raw honey to help with the taste. Drink this and find a comfortable spot to take a nap. When you wake up, drink more water then take it easy until you feel like yourself again.

### SPICY HANGOVER TEA

Cayenne and lemon tea can recharge the body while you are recovering from a hangover. One of the best things about cayenne is that it is a natural pain reliever, so if you are suffering from a headache, it can help bring relief. Cayenne also calms an upset stomach caused by overindulgence in alcohol. The addition of lemon helps to create a more alkaline state in the body that may be offset by drinking alcohol. It can also help relieve any headache or body pains you may be experiencing as you recover.

Many people assume that drinking something spicy would upset the stomach when it is already upset from a hangover. However, the truth is that cayenne can calm an upset stomach and bring relief. Gently stir one half teaspoon of ground cayenne into three fourths cup of hot water. When it is fully dissolved, add one fourth of a cup of lemon juice. Finally, add a teaspoon of raw honey. This will create a surprisingly pleasant drink to help ease any bodily distress.

## Headache

### COOLING HEADACHE TEA

For a cooling and refreshing tea that works to melt tension and reduce inflammation, combine soothing linden flower with yarrow. Linden flowers help to ease tension in the body and mind, which often contributes to headaches. Yarrow has the unique ability to lower inflammation in the head that causes restrictions on blood vessels. When these blood vessels are restricted, a headache can result. Together, yarrow and linden flowers work to get rid of a headache on different levels. Try infusing one teaspoon each of linden flowers and yarrow (leaves and flowers) in one cup of hot water for seven to ten minutes. Allow this to completely cool and drink it on ice for invigorating relief. Drink 1 to 3 cups of this cooling headache tea as needed for tension headaches or headaches caused by inflammation.

### WARMING HEADACHE TEA

Cayenne and ginger pair perfectly in a warming tea that can ease pain and knock out a headache. Cayenne is famous for its analgesic qualities and ginger is equally known for its ability to reduce pain and inflammation. Oftentimes, inflammation is to blame for a headache because it restricts blood flow in the head. Cayenne can help to restore circulation while ginger works to reduce inflammation, helping blood flow return to normal. Cayenne is a source of a compound called capsaicin, which is useful for activating nerve cells to reduce pain. Infuse one teaspoon of finely chopped or grated ginger (dried or fresh) with one half of a teaspoon of ground cayenne in one cup of hot water. Allow these to infuse for five to seven minutes. Stir the tea well to help the cayenne powder dissolve into the water. Consume one cup of this tea as needed to reduce pain from a headache.

### PEPPERY HEADACHE TEA

Black pepper is another spicy herb that can help with pain from a headache. This is because it contains compounds that are both anti-inflammatory and analgesic. In addition, a tea made with black pepper can help calm an upset stomach caused by a migraine or headache. To make this tea, infuse one teaspoon of organic black peppercorns into one cup of hot water for five to seven minutes. For an extra anti-inflammatory and analgesic kick, try adding one teaspoon of chopped (fresh or dried) turmeric root. Both black pepper and turmeric complement one another. Black pepper can also help the body better absorb the medicinal compounds in turmeric. Drink one to two cups of this tea as needed for respite from a headache or migraine.

## SOOTHING HEADACHE TEA

Valerian and chamomile aren't just great for helping you relax. They also have analgesic, anti-inflammatory, and anti-spasmodic properties. This tea blend is perfect for headaches caused by anxiety, stress or other nerve issues. It can help to relax the body, relieve tension, and ease any pain in the body. It will also help you sleep off a particularly bad headache or migraine. This is best taken at the first sign of a headache or migraine. When you feel one coming on, infuse a teaspoon of chopped valerian root and a teaspoon of chamomile flowers in one cup of hot water for seven to ten minutes. Consume this and find a peaceful, dark location to take a nap or just close your eyes and meditate for a while.

## *Heartburn/Reflux/GERD*

### MARSHMALLOW INFUSION

Marshmallow root may be just what you need to help soothe an irritated throat or esophagus. It can also help negate the acidity of the contents of the stomach, bringing much needed relief to those with heartburn or acid reflux. To make an effective infusion, start by bringing two cups of water to boil on the stove. Meantime, fill a glass jar with two tablespoons of dried marshmallow root. Carefully pour the boiling water over the marshmallow root and let this infuse for two to four hours. You want to see the liquid become somewhat thicker and attain a "smooth" consistency. After two to four hours, consume this in half-cup increments throughout the day to support an alkaline stomach and prevent or treat heartburn and reflux.

### PREVENTATIVE BITTER TINCTURE

Bitter herbs are herbs that aid in digestion and help to calm a wide variety of stomach and digestive issues. They are also perfect for daily use to prevent heartburn, acid reflux, and gastroesophageal reflux disease (GERD). Some bitter alkaline herbs include dandelion root/leaf and burdock root. These herbs are also rich sources of vitamins and minerals the body needs to stay healthy. Mugwort is another digestive bitter and can ease indigestion, bloating, gas, and more. Combine these in a tincture for a powerful way to prevent and treat a wide range of digestive discomforts. Fill a sterile glass jar with one part dandelion leaf and root, one part mugwort, and one part burdock root. Next, completely cover the plant material with at least 80 proof alcohol. Let this sit and infuse for four to six weeks, shaking the bottle daily to help it infuse better. After 4 - 6 weeks, strain out the tincture and bottle the liquid in a dropper bottle. Take two droppers full daily, spacing doses out by taking one in the morning and one in the evening. Take each dose with a little food and make sure you drink plenty of water to keep healthy and encourage proper digestion.

### QUICK-ACTING HEARTBURN TEA

For quick relief from heartburn, try making a strong tea with sage. Sage can help negate acid and calm an upset stomach. It is also carminative and aids in digestion. Infuse two teaspoons of fresh or dried sage leaves into one cup of hot water for seven to ten minutes. Drink one to two cups as needed for quick relief from heartburn. Make sure to avoid foods and drinks that can trigger heartburn like tomatoes, orange juice, alcohol, onions, garlic, or spicy foods.

### Soothing Heartburn Tea

Chamomile and catnip work together to soothe an irritated esophagus while reducing inflammation and settling an upset stomach. They are also perfect for calming stress or anxiety that can trigger heartburn. Combine one teaspoon each of chamomile and catnip and infuse them in one cup of hot water for five to seven minutes. Drink this tea as needed when you need relief from stress or anxiety-induced heartburn.

## Indigestion/Dyspepsia

### Pre-Emptive Bitter Tincture

Mugwort and dandelion are great together in a bitter tincture for preventing indigestion if you are prone to indigestion after meals. If you take this tincture before and after eating, it can help prevent issues before they have a chance to emerge. Combine one part dandelion leaf, one part dandelion root, and one part mugwort in a glass jar. Next, completely cover the plant material with at least 80 proof alcohol. Allow this to sit and infuse for four to six weeks, making sure you store it in a cool, dark place. Shake the bottle daily to get the plant material to infuse in the alcohol quicker. After 4 - 6 weeks, strain out the liquid and bottle it. Take one to two droppers full before and after each meal. Drink plenty of water and avoid overeating. Avoid foods that trigger indigestion like spicy or fried foods.

### Carminative Tincture

Chamomile and sage pair well in a tincture to settle an upset stomach and promote digestive health. Chamomile soothes and settles the stomach while sage treats and prevents discomforts like gas, bloating, and indigestion. Combine one part sage leaves and one part chamomile flowers in a glass jar and completely cover them with at least 80 proof alcohol. Let this infuse for four to six weeks before straining out. Store the tincture in a dropper bottle and take one to three droppers full as needed to settle the stomach and calm any indigestion, gas, bloating, or digestive discomfort.

### Digestive Tea

Chickweed and stinging nettle work seamlessly in this tea blend to promote healthy digestion and flush out toxins that lead to problems like infections and diarrhea. Chickweed is often used to soothe and treat skin issues because it is highly anti-inflammatory and cooling. However, it is also a nutritious edible herb that can heal the body when taken internally. Stinging nettle is a diuretic and can help the body get rid of excess water, sending it out through the bowels or urine. This flushes out unwanted toxins in the digestive and urinary tract. Combine one teaspoon each of fresh chickweed and fresh or dried stinging nettle leaves. Infuse these in one cup of hot water for five to seven minutes before consuming. Drink one cup daily for digestive maintenance.

## STRONG DIGESTIVE TEA

Ginger, fennel, and catnip make a strong combination for those wishing for a strong remedy to get rid of digestive woes like gas, bloating, upset stomach, and indigestion. These herbs help promote healthy digestion and support the gentle elimination of the bowels. Ginger is anti-inflammatory, making it ideal for calming any digestive issues that lead to inflammation. Fennel is highly carminative and aids in digestion. Catnip is soothing and nourishing to the digestive tract. Combine one teaspoon each of grated ginger, fennel seeds, and catnip leaves. Infuse these in a cup of hot water for ten to fifteen minutes to create a stronger tea for treating digestive ailments. Drink one to two cups daily as needed for digestive health.

## QUICK-ACTING DIGESTIVE TEA

Prodigiosa acts fast to calm issues of the digestive system such as diarrhea, stomach pain, and indigestion. Lupulo complements prodigiosa well because it works to calm the body and mind, easing tension and anxiety that leads to digestive issues. Lupulo is carminative, sedative, and anti-inflammatory. Create a tea to rapidly banish digestive woes by combining one teaspoon of dried prodigiosa and one teaspoon of dried lupulo and infusing these in one cup of hot water for ten minutes. Drink one cup as needed for timely relief.

## Insomnia

## END-OF-THE-DAY ELIXIR

At the end of a long day, it can be difficult to shut off a racing mind and get ready for sleep. A gentle elixir that helps get the brain ready for sleep can help you get the rest you need. This elixir is made with blue vervain and skullcap. Blue vervain acts on the nerves to settle the body and help rein in the mind. Skullcap is a powerful nervine that can ease the nerves and calm frustration, anxiety, stress, and a feeling of being overwhelmed. This elixir will help you reset to take on the next day. Combine one part blue vervain and one part skullcap in a glass jar. Cover half of the plant material with brandy and half with at least 80 proof alcohol. Sit the jar somewhere to infuse for four to six weeks. After four to six weeks are up, strain out the liquid. Add a teaspoon or two of raw honey for taste if desired and shake well. Take one to three droppers full at the end of the day as you are preparing to go to bed. At least one hour before bed time, avoid all screens from phones, tablets, or televisions. Blue light from these screens can mess with the brain and keep the body awake longer.

## SLEEP FORMULA

Lupulo, valerian, and lemon balm combine in this powerful sleep formula to help you get to sleep fast and stay asleep. If you have trouble getting to sleep or wake up in the night restless and unable to get back to sleep, this formula is for you. Lupulo is a mild sedative and can help relax the body and mind. Valerian is one of the most effective sleep remedies for its effect on the Central Nervous System. Lemon balm is a nervine herb that can bring peace and quiet to an overwhelmed mind. Combine one part each of dried and chopped valerian roots, lupulo, and lemon balm in a glass jar. Completely cover the contents of the jar with at least 80 proof alcohol. Let this sit in a cool, dark place for four to six weeks, shaking it daily to help it infuse. After 4 - 6 weeks, strain out the liquid and bottle it in a dropper bottle. Take two to three droppers full anywhere from thirty minutes to one hour before bedtime. At bedtime, take another two to three droppers full of this formula. If you happen to wake up in the night and find yourself in the same situation where you cannot fall back asleep, take two droppers full again. Before bedtime, avoid looking at blue light from screens to help your brain prepare for sleep. Try doing a relaxing activity, like soaking in a warm bath with Epsom salt. Make it a point to get a good night's sleep and set regular and consistent bedtimes.

### INSOMNIA RELIEF TEA

Linden flower is a wonderful alkaline herb for insomnia because it is sedative and calming.

It pairs great with California poppy because California poppy is nervine and helps with minor aches and pains as well. Together, these potent flowers create a tea that helps to bring on sleep naturally and ease the body and mind. Combine one teaspoon each of California poppy and linden flower in a tea bag and infuse this in very hot water for five to seven minutes. Drink one to two cups of this tea around one hour prior to bedtime. Unwind with an activity such as meditation or a warm bath after drinking this tea.

### SWEET DREAMS TEA

Chamomile and lavender have been utilized for thousands of years to help with sleep issues, as well as anxiety, stress, and nerve issues. They are also gentle enough to be enjoyed by children and adults alike. Chamomile's anti-spasmodic properties come in handy when helping the body get to sleep. It can also help settle the mind. Lavender helps calm the body and slow things down a bit. It is especially useful if you are frustrated, agitated, or overwhelmed. Combine one teaspoon of chamomile flowers and one teaspoon of lavender buds in a tea bag and infuse this in hot water for five to seven minutes. Drink 1 to 3 cups of this sweet dreams tea around one hour before bedtime. Chamomile and lavender also pair well when used in aromatherapy. If you have a diffuser and essential oils, try diffusing five drops of chamomile and five drops of lavender in your room at bedtime to expedite sleep.

## Menstrual Cycle Irregularities

### STEADY CYCLE TEA

By far, one of the best herbs for balancing the hormones and fixing issues that lead to menstrual irregularities is vitex, or chaste tree berry. This berry is an adaptogen, meaning it is a special type of herb that brings balance to whatever is out of balance in the body. It can target the cause and work to bring healing and restoration. Some adaptogenic herbs target the immune system or energy levels in the body, but chaste tree berry targets hormone abnormalities in women specifically. Whether the issue is with high estrogen, progesterone, or prolactin levels, chaste tree berry can help get the levels where they need to be so you can have a normal menstrual cycle.

After taking chaste tree berry for several months steadily, you may begin to notice that your menstrual cycles are right on time and not as painful as they once were. It does need to be taken on a regular basis and for several months before you begin to notice a change.

However, once you begin to notice a difference, you will feel much better emotionally and physically. Drink a tea made with chaste tree berries daily for best results. Infuse one teaspoon of dried chaste tree berries in one cup of very hot water for seven to ten minutes. Add some raw honey to taste, as chaste tree berries can be bitter depending on how potent they are. You may not notice a change right away, but keep drinking this tea and give the berries a chance to change your hormones for the better.

## BLEED ON TEA

A menstrual cycle should come each month, optimally every twenty eight days. A regular cycle is a sign of health and hormonal balance. If you start to notice a change in your menstrual cycles, this could be a sign you need to look into your hormone levels. If your cycles are getting farther and farther apart, you might look into drinking the chaste tree berry tea daily (as detailed above). If your cycle still hasn't come and you know for sure you are not pregnant, you can try bringing it one with contribo. This alkaline herb has been utilized for centuries for its emmenagogue properties. Try infusing one teaspoon of contribo into one cup of hot water for ten to fifteen minutes. Drink one cup of this daily until your cycle begins. Begin drinking chaste tree berry tea daily to manage this as well.

## DAILY SOOTHING MENSTRUAL TEA

Raspberry Leaf is a nourishing uterine tonic. These leaves can help tone the uterus and keep it healthy. Stinging nettle is a highly nutritious alkaline herb that can provide the body with the nutrients it needs to stay healthy with balanced hormones. When combined in a tea, these two herbs work well for maintaining menstrual and uterine health. Infuse one teaspoon each of dried red raspberry leaf and stinging nettle into one cup of hot water for five to seven minutes before consuming. Drink one cup of this daily for a healthy menstrual cycle.

## Nausea and Vomiting

## CALMING TEA

Chamomile and nettle can work together in a tea for calming the nerves, as well as nausea that may be interfering with your life. Chamomile's aroma is enough for some people to quell nausea. It is anti-spasmodic and helps settle spasms that lead to vomiting. Nettle can help replace lost nutrients if you have been vomiting. Combine one teaspoon of dried chamomile flowers and one teaspoon of dried stinging nettle leaves in a tea bag and infuse this in hot water for seven to ten minutes. Put a small amount of raw honey to taste. Drink one to three cups of this tea as needed to manage nausea and vomiting, as well as to calm the body and ease stress.

## GINGER EMERGENCY FORMULA

Ginger is an excellent herb for reducing nausea and vomiting. Just the scent alone can help stave off nausea. Ginger can settle an upset stomach and reduce gastrointestinal discomfort. Combining ginger with peppermint is one of the best known remedies for managing nausea. Peppermint is naturally carminative and helps ease digestive woes. Its light, invigorating scent is uplifting and can eliminate nausea. Peppermint blends well with ginger both aromatically and in formulas for nausea. Try combining one part peppermint leaves and one part chopped ginger root in a glass jar. Pour alcohol over the plant material, covering it at least three-fourths of the way. Top the rest off with raw honey. Shake the bottle well to help it blend. Store this somewhere in a cool, dark place to infuse for four to six weeks. After four to six weeks are up, strain out the liquid through a strainer and bottle it. Take five milliliters of this formula as needed to eradicate nausea, an upset stomach, gas, bloating, and other digestive discomforts.

## *Rash*

### DRY RASH SALVE

For rashes that are inflamed, red, irritated, and dry, try a soothing salve made with chickweed. Chickweed is one of the most effective herbs for calming the skin. It provides a cooling sensation that helps to lessen irritation and provide relief. The addition of calendula flowers makes this salve extra effective and healing. Calendula is known for its skin-healing properties. It is soothing, healing, and regenerating. Infuse one part chickweed and one part calendula in a carrier oil (jojoba is good for this type of rash). Let this sit in a cool, dark place for four to six weeks to infuse, or you can infuse faster with heat. If you want to make this rash salve faster, you can put your plants in the carrier oil like normal and then place the jar of oil and plants (make sure its glass) in a pan of hot water on the stove for up to twelve hours. Make sure the heat is not turned up to high; this is best infused under low heat for an extended period of time. After the plant material has successfully infused, strain out the oil. In a double boiler, add eight ounces of chickweed and calendula-infused oil and one ounce of beeswax. Let this sit under low heat in the double boiler until the beeswax has completely melted. Stir the beeswax and oil together well. If you wish, you may add ten to fifteen drops of lavender essential oil (or any other skin-soothing oil) to the mixture. Pour this into jars to cool and it will take on a thicker, salve-like consistency. This salve is perfect for application on the skin because it is not runny. It stays in place so it can heal the area faster. Apply it as often as needed to rashes.

### WEEPY RASH POULTICE

Weepy rashes are often the result of contact with something that causes a reaction. For example, poisonous plants like poison ivy are known to cause a weepy rash that itches fiercely. For these rashes, you will need a plant that is soothing, healing, and promotes drying of the rash. One of the most popular plants for treating weepy rashes is jewelweed. It is a very common plant found along creeks and wet areas throughout North America. It is often found growing in abundance in the summertime. It is distinguished by its "jewel-like" red and orange flowers hanging from the plant like a necklace. Legend has it that jewelweed grows where poison ivy grows because nature knows what we need to heal. The inner stems have a gel-like substance that is somewhat reminiscent to aloe vera. It makes the perfect poultice because of this. Mash up jewelweed stems until you have a nice poultice. Apply this directly to the affected area as often as needed to treat a weepy rash. Harvest enough jewelweed to make multiple poultices so you can keep treating the rash until it heals.

## SKIN-SOOTHING TEA

Treat skin from the inside out with a tea that promotes healthy skin. One of the most popular plants for beautiful skin is rose. This is because it is gently astringent and emollient. Rose is also wonderful in tea and can be consumed to promote healthy skin. In addition to rose, hibiscus flowers have been used traditionally to treat skin issues. Hibiscus is also hydrating to dull skin, giving it a glow and vibrancy. Hibiscus and rose combine perfectly in a tea for skin health. Combine one teaspoon of dried rose petals with one teaspoon of dried hibiscus flower and infuse this into one cup of hot water for five to seven minutes. Tea made from these flowers will turn a gorgeous pink color. Drink one to two cups a day to promote healthy skin. It is said that beauty begets beauty, so it is no wonder such beautiful flowers make the skin beautiful.

## RASH WASH

For a calming wash to treat a variety of rashes, try a wash made with chickweed, chamomile, and witch hazel. Chickweed works to treat inflammation and irritation, chamomile works to reduce redness and heal angry skin, and witch hazel's astringent properties work to tighten, tone, and heal skin tissue. Together, these three powerful herbs can cleanse and heal a rash fast. Start by boiling two cups of water on the stove. Fill a glass jar with one teaspoon each of chickweed, chamomile, and witch hazel bark. Carefully pour the water over the plant material in the jar and let this infuse for one to two hours. When it has completely cooled, wash the affected areas with this liquid thoroughly. You can also soak a clean cloth in this to apply to the rash to further promote healing after you wash the area well. Refrigerate what you don't use. This will keep in the refrigerator for up to three days, so make sure you use it up within this time period, treating the rash often.

## *Sinusitis/Stuffy Nose*

### SINUS-CLEARING STEAM BATH

A steamy bath is a very effective way to break up stubborn mucous in the sinuses and reduce congestion. The addition of eucalyptus leaves can help release oils that further work to open the airways and prevent infection in the sinus area. Treat yourself to a soothing eucalyptus bath by running hot water (as hot as you can stand). Shut the curtain or door to trap in steam. Place one half cup of dried and crumbled eucalyptus leaves in a muslin bag. Shut the bag well and place it in the bath water to soak and infuse. Get in the bath and soak as long as you can, practicing deep breathing techniques to better inhale the healing eucalyptus steam. Do this as needed to treat and prevent sinus issues.

### SINUS-RELIEVING TEA

For a tea to treat sinus infections and mucous in the sinus area, try utilizing a combination of sage and pau d' arco bark. Sage is an expectorant and can help to get mucous out of the body. It is also antimicrobial, that's why it can help treat any infection in the sinuses. Pau d' arco is is highly antimicrobial and has antibiotic properties that work to target any infection before it causes problems in the body. Together, sage and pau d' arco can effectively treat and prevent sinus infections. When the sinuses are congested, the trapped mucous in the sinus cavities can begin to grow bacteria that leads to infection. Fevers, chills, and serious headaches in the sinus area can develop as a result. This tea can help take care of these issues before they get serious. Infuse one teaspoon each of pau d' arco bark and sage leaves into one cup of hot water for seven to ten minutes. Drink one to two cups daily to release trapped mucous and kill infection-causing germs in the sinuses.

## Mucous-Freeing Tea

To break up mucous, try a combination of mullein and pleurisy root. Mullein is a known herbal demulcent and expectorant. Pleurisy root is also expectorant and is used to target mucous and fluid in the airways. Pleurisy root is a very common "weed" found throughout North America. It often goes by the name "butterfly weed" because butterflies love this pollinator. It has bright red-orange flowers that bloom in the summer. The root of this plant is what is used medicinally, so make sure if you harvest any to leave some as well. Combine one teaspoon of dried and chopped mullein leaves with one teaspoon of dried and chopped pleurisy root in a tea bag. Infuse this into a cup of very hot water for seven to ten minutes before consuming. Drink one to three cups daily to release mucous and fluid in the sinuses, bronchial area, and lungs.

## *Sore Throat*

## Sore Throat Tea

Wild Bergamot, or "bee balm" as it is sometimes called, was used extensively by indigenous people in North America to treat a sore throat. This powerful plant was introduced to settlers who were astounded at its effectiveness. Studies show wild bergamot to be highly antimicrobial and potent. It has a chemical profile similar to thyme. Another native North American plant that was used in conjunction with wild bergamot is Echinacea. There are several medicinal species of Echinacea throughout North America, but one of the most studied species is Echinacea purpurea. Echinacea has been shown in multiple studies to have antiviral, antiseptic, and anti-inflammatory properties. It has been used for everything from a sore throat to boosting the immune system to prevent sickness. Combining wild bergamot with Echinacea will help boost the immune system to fight off any germs responsible for the sore throat. Combine one teaspoon of dried and chopped Echinacea (all parts of the plant are used) and one teaspoon of dried and chopped wild bergamot aerial parts. Infuse this in a cup of hot water for seven to ten minutes. Consume one to three cups daily to treat a sore throat, strep throat, or any other throat infection.

## Herbal Gargle

Pau d' arco is one of the best alkaline plants for treating a sore throat caused by the streptococcus infection. Its strong antibiotic properties target the bacteria and kill it, restoring health and bringing relief. The addition of herbs like sage and yarrow help to cleanse, soothe, and heal affected tissues in the throat. To make a gargle with these plants, start by bringing one cup of water to boil on the stove. Add one teaspoon each of pau d' arco, sage, and yarrow. Bring the heat down and let these infuse for fifteen minutes. Add a teaspoon of sea salt or Himalayan salt and let this dissolve well. Strain out the liquid and let it cool completely. Measure out one half ounce of this liquid and gargle it for one to two minutes, making sure to get the liquid to the back of the throat as you gargle. Spit this out and repeat up to five times daily to treat a throat infection. Drink the "Sore Throat Tea" detailed above for even faster healing.

## THROAT-SOOTHING TEA

Sometimes a sore throat can feel extremely uncomfortable and make it hard to swallow. This affects eating and drinking, leading to poor health and dehydration. If you find that you have a sore throat that makes it difficult to swallow, try a combination of chamomile and chaparral for relief. Chamomile calms the surface tissue as much as it calms the mind. It can soothe the area, while reducing inflammation. Chaparral is highly anti-inflammatory, helping to bring down inflammation in the throat that leads to pain and discomfort. Combine one teaspoon each of chaparral and chamomile in a tea bag and infuse this in hot water for five to seven minutes. Add one to three teaspoons of raw honey to help further soothe the throat, as well as kill bacteria that may be causing the sore throat. Drink one to two cups daily for soothing relief.

## FRUITY GARGLE

Elderberry isn't just great for treating a virus and boosting the immune system. It is also a powerfully anti-inflammatory fruit. It can relieve a sore throat effectively, while also reducing any drainage that may be causing irritation in the throat. Red raspberry leaf is a mild astringent and can help tighten and tone the throat tissues, relieving soreness and pain. Its astringent properties are the result of tannins in the leaves. Herbs with tannins have traditionally been used to treat inflamed tissues both internally and externally. A combination of elderberry and red raspberry leaves make a fruity and delicious way to treat a sore throat! To make this gargle, start by boiling two cups of water on the stove. Add one tablespoon each of dried and crumbled red raspberry leaves and dried elderberries. Lower the heat and let this simmer until the liquid is reduced by half. You should have one cup of liquid when you are finished. Strain out the liquid and add two tablespoons of raw honey. Stir it in well until it is completely dissolved. Let the gargle cool completely before use. Gargle one half ounce of this liquid for two minutes as needed for relief from a sore throat. Refrigerate the gargle and continue using it as needed until it is gone.

## SWEET COUGH DROPS

Does a nasty cough and congestion have your throat sore and inflamed? Too much coughing can really irritate the throat tissues, resulting in tenderness and pain. Ginger and sage combine in this remedy to bring relief fast. For a soothing, antitussive treatment, start by boiling two cups of water on the stove. Add two tablespoons each of dried and chopped ginger and sage. Reduce heat and let this simmer until the liquid is reduced by half. Carefully strain out the liquid and clean out the pot. Add the herb-infused liquid back to the pot under medium heat. Add one to one-and-a-half cups of raw honey and stir everything until it is well-blended. Bring this back to a boil and keep it boiling until the honey and water mixture begins to thicken. When you are able to take small amounts on a spoon and place them on wax paper and they do not run, but rather harden, this is when you know it is ready. Be very careful because this honey mixture is very hot and can burn the skin easily. Keep taking small spoonful's of the mixture and dropping them onto the wax paper. Leave them to harden fully. You can speed up this process by putting your sheets of wax paper in the refrigerator for several hours. When they are fully hard, sprinkle them with powdered cinnamon, ginger, or turmeric to add additional medicinal power while preventing them from sticking together in a container. Take these tasty drops as needed to help with a cough or sore throat.

## Sprains and Strains

### SOFT TISSUE INJURY LINIMENT

For sprains, one of the best herbs to reduce inflammation and tighten stretched ligaments and/or tendons is Solomon's seal. This native North American plant has been used traditionally for inflammation and trauma. It almost works like an adaptogenic herb with its ability to tighten or loosen, depending on what the body needs. The root of this plant is used in herbal remedies, both externally and internally. Always harvest this plant mindfully, as it is not common in some areas. Harvest the roots, clean them, and chop them well. Lay them to dry. When they are completely dry, fill a clean glass jar with the root pieces. Cover them completely in a carrier oil. Let this sit and infuse for four to six weeks in a cool, dark place. Strain out the oil and add eight ounces of it to a double boiler. Next, add one ounce of beeswax pellets. Heat this gently until the beeswax melts, making sure to stir continually. Pour this into small jars to cool. Apply a liberal amount as needed to injured joints or areas of the body that have sustained trauma.

### TOPICAL PAIN RELIEF

Arnica is a flower known for its ability to ease pain, especially when it comes to pain from injured joints. Historically, it has been a major ingredient in an oil infusion called "trauma oil." Trauma oil is created using several different plants in addition to arnica. These include St. John's Wort, known for helping nerve pain and inflammation, and calendula flowers, known for soothing and calming. Infusing all three of these flowers in olive oil creates a powerful topical pain relief remedy. Fill a jar with one part calendula, one part arnica, and one part St. John's Wort flowers. If possible, it is best to use fresh or wilted St. John's Wort flowers. Cover the flowers completely with a good quality olive oil and let this infuse for four to six weeks before straining it out. Shake your jar daily to help the flowers infuse better. Strain out the oil and bottle it in a tinted jar to keep sunlight from degrading it. Label it and store it in a cool, dark place to use as needed. Apply a liberal amount to affected areas as often as you can to promote healing, lower inflammation, and reduce pain. Any time you are working with arnica, be sure to keep it out of open wounds. This includes cuts and scrapes. Arnica is fine for the skin and very effective at what it does, but it should not get into the bloodstream or it could cause issues.

### QUICK-ACTING PAIN RELIEF

For quick pain relief from the swelling and trauma associated with sprains and related injuries, try a twofold approach: First, apply a large cabbage leaf to the affected area. Cabbage leaves work quickly to lower inflammation and reduce pain. You may remove and reapply a new leaf as needed. Next, take two droppers-full of a tincture made with white willow bark. Repeat this every two to three hours as needed for pain. White willow contains a compound called salicin that specifically targets pain and inflammation in the body. This compound is still used today to create over-the-counter pain relievers like aspirin. However, taking white willow tincture doesn't affect the kidneys or gut like aspirin. To create this tincture, shave off the inner bark of the white willow tree. Fill a jar with shavings and completely cover them in at least 80 proof alcohol. Let this infuse for four to six weeks and then strain out the liquid. Store your tincture in a cool, dark place to use for pain relief.

## SWEET RELIEF TEA

A tea made with chamomile and linden flowers can help provide relief from pain, while promoting relaxation and reducing any stress related to pain. Combine one teaspoon of linden flowers with one teaspoon of chamomile flowers in a tea bag and infuse this in one cup of hot water for five to seven minutes. Add a small amount of raw honey to taste and enjoy a cup of this soothing tea up to three times daily for relief from pain from sprains, muscle aches, joint aches, and even headaches.

## *Stress*

## RESCUE ELIXIR

For an elixir that comes to the rescue to calm the body and mind, blue vervain is a true friend. Blue vervain calms the nerves and promotes relaxation quickly. Create a strong but sweet extract with blue vervain by filling a jar with the aerial parts of the plant. Cover them three-fourths of the way with at least 80 proof alcohol and the rest of the way with raw honey or brandy. Shake this well each day and store it in a cool, dark place to infuse. After four to six weeks, strain out your elixir and take two to three droppers full when you are feeling overwhelmed, stressed, or anxious. Do this up to three times daily.

## SOOTHE UP TEA

Always there to help soothe the body and provide relief, linden flowers can be an ally for stress and stress-related issues. If you find yourself in need of some serious soothing, try infusing one teaspoon of linden flowers into one cup of hot water for five to seven minutes. Add raw honey to taste. Drink one to five cups of this tasty tea daily for management of stress.

## NERVE SOOTHING TEA

For herbs that work specifically on the nerves, try a tea made with skullcap and valerian root. Skullcap is a wonderful herb for combating frustration, anxiousness, and the feeling of being "on-edge." Valerian is a powerful nervine that helps to relax the nerves, muscles, and mind. Combining these two nervine herbs is sure to soothe aggravated nerves. Start by adding one teaspoon each of dried skullcap (aerial parts) and dried and chopped valerian root to a tea bag. Infuse this into one cup of very hot water for seven to ten minutes. Drink one to three cups as needed to soothe the nerves and find relief.

## CALMING TEA

Lavender and lupulo can help calm you down when you need it most. Lavender boasts the ability to calm the body and has even been shown in studies to lower blood pressure. This is an important attribute since stress and anxiety almost always raise blood pressure. Lupulo, or hops, is a nervine and sedative plant that help quiet a racing mind and relax the body. Combine one teaspoon of dried lavender buds and one teaspoon of hops in a tea bag and infuse this in a cup of hot water for five to ten minutes. (Let it sit for the full ten minutes for a stronger tea). Drink one to three cups of this tea daily to manage stress and help pacify the body so it can stay healthy and function properly.

### Shake-It-Off Tea

Chamomile has been associated with stress relief for centuries, and it is still used today to help reduce stress and anxiety. Motherwort is a gentle and helpful herb for stress as well. It is also great for heart health and lowering blood pressure. It can provide quick relief from tension and nervous conditions. Both chamomile and motherwort complement each other and taste great together in a tea for stress. Combine one teaspoon each of chamomile flowers and motherwort (aerial parts) in a tea bag. Let this infuse in one cup of hot water for seven to ten minutes before enjoying. Try drinking one to two cups for times when you feel overwhelmed or nervous.

## Wounds

### Wound Wash

The first step for wound care is to wash a wound well. This may very well be one of the most important things you can do to treat a wound correctly. Yarrow makes an excellent wound wash because of its strong antiseptic properties. It is also helps promote healing for the wound. Make a simple wound wash with the aerial parts of the yarrow plant by infusing two teaspoons of dried yarrow in one cup of hot water for fifteen to twenty minutes. When this has completely cooled, strain it out and wash the wound with it. Repeat this prior to treating with a salve or ointment as often as possible to help a wound heal fast. Consider applying raw honey to the wound after washing it with yarrow because the honey can help kill dangerous bacteria and promote recovery.

### Pine Resin Salve

Pine resin is another great wound remedy because it contains antimicrobial properties that help cleanse and heal a wound. The prevention of infection is key to getting a wound to heal properly, and pine resin is perfect for this task. Pine trees have been used medicinally for generations because many parts of the tree benefit humans. For example, the needles have been used traditionally to treat scurvy and are a good source of vitamin C. The needles are also steam distilled into an essential oil to help open the airways and promote respiratory health. The resin is the substance the tree produces when it has a wound. The tree tries to "heal" its own wound by covering the area with this sticky substance. Pine resin can be collected from the pine three where there is a missing limb or abrasion. Only if completely necessary should you drill a small hole to collect the resin. Visit your pine trees daily to collect resin until you have at least one tablespoon. You may need a knife or object to scrape the sap from the tree if it has ran down the trunk. In a double boiler, add the pine resin to eight ounces of a healing carrier oil like olive oil or emu oil. Let this melt together gently until the pine resin is no longer in chunks. Add one ounce of beeswax and allow this to melt into the oil. Stir under low heat until everything is blended together sufficiently. Remove the mixture from heat. At this time, you may consider adding ten to twenty drops of a wound-healing essential oil like tea tree or lavender. Pour the salve into jars to cool. Apply to wounds after washing them to promote restoration of any skin trauma.

## TOPICAL APPLICATION FOR ABRASIONS

Yarrow and chickweed work perfectly in a salve to target several issues related to wound healing. For starters, yarrow prevents infection and stops bleeding. Chickweed comes to the rescue for angry, irritated skin that has been agitated by a wound. It works to cool and soothe the skin while repairing any damage. Infuse one part chickweed (wilted or dried) and one part yarrow in a carrier oil for four to six weeks, shaking it daily. Keep your herb infusion in a cool, dark place during this time. Strain out the oil after four to six weeks. You may choose to treat abrasions by using this oil alone or combining eight ounces of the oil with one ounce of beeswax in a double boiler for a salve that has a thicker consistency. Apply this to abrasions as needed (after washing) to mend the skin and keep bacteria at bay.

## TOPICAL WASH FOR CUTS

For cuts, especially ones that seem to have a hard time with blood clotting, try a wash made with yarrow and shepherd's purse. This wash works to cleanse a wound, stop bleeding, and repair the broken skin. Infuse two teaspoons each of dried yarrow and shepherd's purse into one cup of hot water for fifteen to twenty minutes. Strain out the liquid and allow it to cool completely. Apply a liberal amount of this wash to cuts and minor lacerations prior to treatment with a salve or raw honey. You can also soak a small clean rag in this wash and apply it to a cut for several minutes to speed up healing and aid in skin renewal.

# REMEDIES FOR COMMON CHILDHOOD PROBLEMS

When it comes to your children's health, you need to know that there are a lot of things that you should be aware of. Keep in mind that it is very easy for a child to get sick especially when they are young since their immune system is not fully developed yet.

There are a lot of ways that you can keep your children as healthy as possible.

You should ensure that your child is given plenty of rest and sleep. It will make a huge difference in their overall health, growth, and development if they get sufficient rest each day. Getting enough sleep also helps improve one's immune system since it allows the body to be fully restored with energy and protect against illness.

Ensure that you wash their hands frequently and always teach them not to touch their mouth with their hands. If they have colds, it would be a good idea to make sure that they are taking medicine or going to the doctor.

You should also make sure that they play outside with friends as opposed to playing video games indoors. This will help them socialize and interact with other people who will keep their immune systems healthy. You should also consider taking your children to a health spa when it is cold because this can help improve their energy levels.

You should make sure that you get your children vaccinated. When it comes to young children, this is very essential since they are still very susceptible to many diseases. Some of the diseases they could contract include rashes, measles, chickenpox, meningitis, and type 1 diabetes. The first three of these diseases can cause quite a lot of harm especially for small children so it is essential to protect against them by giving them proper vaccinations.

The first vaccination that should be given is a triple vaccine, which protects against three diseases. The second vaccine is a combination vaccine and the third one is the meningitis C injection. In most cases, this is enough to help protect your child from these diseases.

It would also be best if you give your children plenty of exercises regularly. That will prevent them from becoming overweight and it will also make their immune system stronger.

1. Echinacea (E. Purpurea)

Echinacea can be taken in liquid form and is most effective when used fresh rather than dry. It should be taken daily for up to 6 months when an immune

boosting remedy is required for best results.

2. Elderberry

This is one of the best natural remedies for colds and flu. Studies have shown that it is effective against a wide range of viruses. For best results, take the elderberry syrup daily during cold and flu season. After six months you can discontinue use as long as symptoms don't frequently recur (when used at appropriate concentration).

3. Garlic

Garlic is an excellent natural remedy for preventing colds, especially during cold and flu season. It has many other benefits as well. Garlic is also an immune stimulant and anti-inflammatory agent. You can take it in capsule form or fresh garlic juice.

4. Ginger

Ginger (Zingiberofficinale) has been used as a medicinal herb for centuries to treat a wide range of ailments such as migraines, sore throats, indigestion, nausea, and the common cold.

For Children Of 0 - 2 Month

1. Newborn Dill [Anethumgraveolens]

This is good for soothing the stomach and its strong anti-inflammatory action promotes fast recovery from ulcers. The same action is seen in ginger. It also has antimicrobial action on bacteria and viruses. Its main active ingredient is anethole which acts as a powerful anti-carcinogen, anti-biotic, anti-fungal, and antiviral agent.

2. Lavender [Lavandulaangustifolia]

Lavender is a very beautiful plant that is widely used in decoration. It has several uses. Its main active ingredients are linalool (a strong antiseptic), linalyl acetate (a potent antimicrobial agent), Lavandula (another natural antibacterial agent), and linalylformate (which has bactericidal effects).

3. Roman Chamomile [Chamaemelumnobile]

The main use of this herb is in the treatment of anxiety and depression.

inflammatory agent. It has the same actions as Lavender and Ginger, but with a stronger antibacterial effect.

4. Yarrow Achilleamillefolium

This herb acts as a powerful anti-carcinogen, anti-biotic, anti-fungal, and antiviral agent. Its active ingredient is yarrow.

5. Elder [Sambucusnigra]

It is now known to have numerous health benefits including its antimicrobial solid action against bacteria, viruses, fungi, and yeasts.

For Children of 2 to12 Months

1. Geranium [Pelargonium Graveolens]

It is good for the stomach, intestines, and lungs. It also helps in improving the immune system. Take Geranium as a herb or as an infusion.

2. Tangerine/Mandarin [Citrus reticulata]

It does not act as a strong antibacterial agent although it has some anti bacterial effects. Nevertheless, a lot of quotes have been made comparing it to lemon water. It can be used in capsules or taken in fresh juice.

3. Eucalyptus [Eucalyptus globules]

It is a very effective anti-bacterial and antifungal agent. It is also an antiviral and antiparasitic agent. It can be taken in the form of capsules or fresh juice.

4. Tea Tree [Melaleuca alternifolia]

Tea tree is a very well-known anti-bacterial, anti-fungal, and antiviral agent. It can be taken in the form of capsules or in fresh juice.

For Children of 12 Months to 5 Years

1. Palmarosa [Cymbopogonmartinii]

This herb is good for the lungs, the spleen, and the liver. It also acts as an anti-cancer agent. It can be taken in capsules or fresh juice.

For Children of 5 Years to 12 Years

1. Clary Sage [Salvia sclerae]

Clary Sage is good for the nervous system, especially the eyes and ears. Its active ingredients are linal-yl acetate, linalool, eugenol (which acts as an antibacterial agent), and beta

caryophyllene (which has antifungal properties).

2. Nutmeg [Myristicafragrans]

This herb is particularly effective against respiratory and digestive tract infections. It is also known to help reduce nausea, vomiting, and diarrhea.

# WHERE TO FIND HERBS GUIDE

Finding fresh herbs can be a tedious task. There are many herbs that can be gathered readily and in huge quantities, but there are others, like thyme and mint, that are very difficult to find. Plus, not all herbs have the same benefits or culinary uses; some might taste better than others, or they might have additional health benefits.

A good herb to know about is borage, which comes from the Latin word "borago", meaning "to refresh." It is a hardy plant that grows almost anywhere, and can actually be planted in containers on your patio or deck. It has a very distinct taste that is similar to cucumber, and it can be used in many recipes. Along with adding a refreshing taste and texture to your food, borage also grows well in areas where most other plants won't thrive. It can also help with digestive problems and sunburn.

The best place to find herbs such as lavender, mint, rosemary or thyme would be a garden store; however these herbs grow easily in home gardens as well. Herbs such as tarragon and dill will only grow well in mild climates, so if you need these for special dishes, it is best to grow them yourself.

One great way to find herbs, such as rosemary or lavender, is to grow them inside your home in small pots. They are easy to care for, and will not spread like most plants. Many of these herbs can also be planted outdoors on a patio or deck where it can get lots of sunlight. Sufficient sunlight is necessary for herbs to thrive without needing to be watered often since they tend to dry out more easily than other plants.

You can also find herbs in many areas of your home. Many kitchens contain more than just the average spice rack, and you can find the herbs that you need there. Such places include: above the stove, in basements, built into a cupboard under the kitchen sink, or even on shelves in closets.

You can purchase many essential oils from a local aromatherapy store as well. Essential oils are non-petroleum based and can be used to keep away insects as well as in healing practices for humans. Many essential oils contain different healing properties such as eucalyptus oil which is known to have an antiseptic quality to it. You can find numerous types of oils in the store and make your own concoctions with them.

Another way to get fresh herbs is to plant them yourself. There are many herbs that grow easily in home gardens and will grow for you, such as oregano, thyme, marjoram and sage.

In order to gather fresh herbs for cooking or use on a day-to-day basis, ones that are most commonly used include: basil, sage, rosemary, oreganoand thyme. These have a very distinct taste that brings a new flavor to almost every dish you eat. Sage is also a good herb to use when you are trying to purify the air and the smell of lavender is very relaxing. Rosemary can be used to help with pain and especially during the cold months when you need something that will heal your sore throat or cracked lips.

The best place to get quality herbs would be in a garden store. They sell various herbs that can be cut or used in other ways such as sauteed with oil for flavor, dried for use in baking or in teas, or simply chopped and sprinkled into food. When buying fresh herbs, try not only to find ones that taste good but also ones that are highly nutritious.

Another way to get fresh herbs would be to plant them yourself. In order to gather fresh herbs for cooking or use on a day-to-day basis, ones that are most commonly used are: basil, sage, rosemary and thyme. These have a very distinct taste that brings a new flavor to almost every dish you eat. Sage is also a good herb to use when you are trying to purify the air and the smell of lavender is very relaxing. Rosemary can be used to help with pain and especially during the cold months when you need something that will heal your sore throat or cracked lips. The best place to get quality herbs would be in a garden store. They sell various herbs that can be cut or used in other ways such as sauteed with oil for flavor, dried for use in baking or in teas, or simply chopped and sprinkled into food. When buying fresh herbs, try not only to find ones that taste good but also ones that are highly nutritious.

Herbs are easy to find all throughout the world, but some of them grow better than others. For example, thyme and rosemary flourish in extremely hot places while mint grows well in cold climates.

When it comes to finding herbs, the best place would be a garden store rather than a regular grocery store because they tend to keep more fresh herbs available for purchase. You can also find herbs in your home, such as on a shelf in the kitchen or even on the counter. You can also easily find herbs in many parts of your home, such as in cupboards under the sink or on a shelf above the stove.

# CONCLUSION

Thank you for choosing this book, and hopefully, it gave you all of the information that you need to know to assist you in getting started on your own path to good health. In this era, while there are lots of viral illnesses everywhere inside the globe, those that are seemed and those that are not but in position. In essence, we must stay guided. What I imply is that understanding the primary arrangements of herbal roots, which might be inner beyond our reach, is critical for our health in a few unspecified times within the destiny even as they want arises. We must take it very intensely for a better, more healthy living for no longer just ourselves, but additionally, our loved ones and own family at massive.

Although this diet completely inhibits protein intake, it surely covers up the required amount of protein from other sources. As any sort of illness or disease arises from mucus accumulation in the human body and level of acidity, it is essential; to maintain these levels in the human body so that it can function properly, and hence it results in longevity. To attain the maximum level of health and well-being, one should get these supplements and follow the diet prescribed by Dr. Sebi. You can start by baby steps towards adopting this lifestyle, and it will shift everything for you in return.

It is essential to maintain an equilibrium in your life regardless of what path you take. Since acidic elements dominate our lifestyle, having an alkaline diet has become more crucial. The excessive use of chemical medicines has further weakened the immune systems of the commoners, making them prone to the complex diseases of today's world. Dr. Sebi worked against this lifestyle, and he enjoyed some severe breakthroughs in his career. If we switch from our current way of life to nature's conduct, we can prevent many diseases and cure others.

The herbal elements that build up Dr. Sebi's diet plan have all the minerals and vitamins vital for our body. His medicines have also shown significant results fighting the diseases, which are considered severe and sometimes untreatable in the medical sciences today with minimum side effects, unlike the chemical treatments of the same subject.

It is easy to heal your body with herbal medicine and the Alkaline Diet by following the few simple rules that Dr. Sebi set out in his guidelines.

- You need to eat alkaline foods regularly as part of your daily diet and try to eat only plant-based foods.
- You need to drink at least one gallon of water every day. This will help keep you hydrated and will also work to flush toxins out of your body that the alkaline foods are releasing.
- You will not be consuming any product that is made from any animal.
- You will not drink alcoholic beverages.

- You will consume the grains that grow naturally as listed in the food list, and you will avoid all products that come from wheat.
- You will not eat fruits that do not have seeds.

Follow these guidelines, eat healthy foods that come from plants, and you will be successful.

And if you found this book enjoyable and it was helpful to you, then a good review on Amazon will be greatly appreciated.

# DOWNLOAD NOW YOUR EBOOKS FOR FREE

# SCAN THE QR CODE AND GET YOUR EBOOKS FOR FREE